Tina Katamea

Newborn screening for sickle cell disease in Lubumbashi

Tina Katamea

Newborn screening for sickle cell disease in Lubumbashi

Assessment of knowledge of the disease, acceptability of neonatal screening and prevalence

Imprint
Any brand names and product names mentioned in this book are subject to trademark, brand or patent protection and are trademarks or registered trademarks of their respective holders. The use of brand names, product names, common names, trade names, product descriptions etc. even without a particular marking in this work is in no way to be construed to mean that such names may be regarded as unrestricted in respect of trademark and brand protection legislation and could thus be used by anyone.

Cover image: www.ingimage.com

This book is a translation from the original published under ISBN 978-620-6-72293-9.

Publisher:
Sciencia Scripts
is a trademark of
Dodo Books Indian Ocean Ltd. and OmniScriptum S.R.L publishing group

120 High Road, East Finchley, London, N2 9ED, United Kingdom
Str. Armeneasca 28/1, office 1, Chisinau MD-2012, Republic of Moldova, Europe
Printed at: see last page
ISBN: 978-620-8-08580-3

TABLE OF CONTENTS

LIST OF PUBLICATIONS

Determining the diagnostic reliability of the Sickle SCAN® rapid test in DND in Lubumbashi, Democratic Republic of Congo

Authors: Tina Katamea, Olivier Mukuku, Oscar N. Luboya, Léon Tshilolo, Stanis O. Wembonyama

Journal : British Journal of Haematology Original article: 2021; 193 (Suppl. 1): 25

Determine the level of acceptability of NHW and the factors influencing it in the city of Lubumbashi in the DRC

Authors: Katamea T, Mukuku O, Mutombo KA, Tshilolo LM, Luboya NO, Wembonyama SO

Journal: Global Journal of Medical, Pharmaceutical, and Biomedical Update

Original article : No GJMPBU_7_2022

Determining the prevalence of sickle cell disease in Lubumbashi, Democratic Republic of Congo

Authors: Tina Katamea, Olivier Mukuku, Stanis O. Wembonyama

Journal: British Journal of Haematology

Original article: 2021; 193 (Suppl. 1): 31

Diagnostic accuracy of the Sickle SCAN® rapid test for newborn screening for sickle cell disease in Lubumbashi, Democratic Republic of Congo

Authors: Tina Katamea, Olivier Mukuku, Oscar N. Luboya, Léon Tshilolo, Stanis O. Wembonyama

Journal: British Journal of Haematology

Original article: 2021; 193 (Suppl. 1): 25

Neonatal screening for sickle cell disease in Lubumbashi, Democratic Republic of Congo: update on the prevalence of the disease

Authors: Tina Katamea, Olivier Mukuku, Stanis O. Wembonyama

Journal: British Journal of Haematology

Original article: 2021; 193 (Suppl. 1): 31

EPIGRAPH

When someone wants to be healthy, we must first ask them if they are prepared to remove the causes of their illness. Only then is it possible to help them.

(Hippocrates)

DEDICATION

To my family,
My parents Paul and Marianne KATAMEA ; My dear husband Didier KAYEYE ;
My children Tina, Marianne, Jérémie, Elie, Elise and David KAYEYE ; My brothers Serge,
Alex, Paul and Marc KATAMEA ;
My sister Ghislaine Isonga ;
My nephews Paul, Sergio, Alex, Paulo, Alino and Alexandre KATAMEA.
I dedicate this work to you.

ACKNOWLEDGEMENTS

My gratitude knows no bounds to the Lord my God, the Almighty, who who has given me the breath of life and the ability to carry out this work.
To my parents Paul and Marianne KATAMEA who have always supported me, accompanied me and gone above and beyond the call of duty right up to the present day, my debt is eternal!

To my dear husband Didier KAYEYE, who was always present and whose support was crucial to the completion of this work. This achievement is a point of arrival of which you can be proud and which you can also consider as your accomplishment.

To the promoter of this work, Professor Emeritus Doctor Stanislas Wembonyama Okitotsho, who, despite his multiple occupations, conducted this thesis with unparalleled commitment and rigour. I will always be as grateful to him as a disciple is to his master. Along with him, I am thinking of all the professors who supported me during the writing of my thesis, namely : Professor Doctor Oscar Luboya Numbi, Professor Doctor André Mutombo Kabamba, Professor Doctor Albert Mwembo Tambwe-A-Nkoy Albert, Professor Doctor Claude Mwamba Mulumba, in addition to their scientific skills, I acquired human values from you that I promise never to betray.

To the medical staff of the NGO LIGHT OF HOPE: Mr Degaul Fikisi, Mr Emil Tambwe. Thank you for your support over the past 5 years.

It was a godsend to benefit from the assistance and solid technical skills of the nursing team in the neonatology department of the Cliniques Universitaires de Lubumbashi.

The success of a project sometimes depends on a few factors that may seem insignificant but are nevertheless decisive. This is the case with the legendary availability of Doctor Dinanga Nzala Patient during the special moments of this thesis, when I was preparing the theoretical part and entering the data collected.

In the same vein, may all the unmentioned heroes in the shadows find in these words the expression of my sincere gratitude.
CT Dr Tina KATAMEA

SUMMARY

Introduction: *Sickle cell disease is an autosomal recessive genetic haemoglobin disorder. It results from a point mutation in the 6th codon of the beta -globin gene (on chromosome 11), followed by the substitution of valine for glutamic acid in the haemoglobin chain. In developing countries, it is often diagnosed late because of the high cost and complexity of conventional diagnostic methods. The aim of this study was to determine the diagnostic reliability of the Sickle SCAN® test in neonatal screening with reference to Hb electrophoresis in Lubumbashi.*

Methodology: *This is a cross-sectional study carried out in several complementary stages depending on the specific objectives.*

The Sickle scan was tested on 365 newborns aged 6 days or less in 9 maternity units; the evaluation of the acceptability of the DND and the factors influencing it were determined in 2032 adults in 7 municipalities; the prevalence of sickle-cell anaemia was determined in 538 newborns aged 6 days or less in 9 maternity units; and healthcare providers' knowledge of sickle-cell anaemia and its DNN was assessed in 465 doctors and nurses working in paediatric settings in 16 health facilities (private and public) in Lubumbashi.

Results: *The reliability of the Sickle scan was 97.26% in the DND; the acceptability of the DND was 84.50% and was influenced by age, sex and religion; the neonatal prevalence of Hb SS was 5.01% and good knowledge of sickle cell disease was 7.96% and 23.66% for the DND.*

Conclusion*: This study has shown that the Sickle scan test is a reliable, beneficial and efficient tool that we recommend for large-scale systematic screening for sickle cell disease in the DRC.*

Key words*: Sickle cell disease, Newborn screening, Reliability, Acceptability, Sickle SCAN®.*

INTRODUCTION

1. Status of the question

Sickle cell anaemia is an autosomal recessive genetic haemoglobin disease. It results from a point mutation in the 6th codon of the beta globin gene (substitution of the amino acid glutamic for valine) on chromosome 11. There are two forms of sickle cell disease; the asymptomatic form found in healthy carriers (AS) does not require medical monitoring but should benefit from genetic counselling, and the symptomatic form manifested by the major sickle cell syndrome (MSC). The latter is made up of SS homozygotes (the most common form) and composite heterozygotes (Sβ thal, SC, SE, etc.) [1]. Every year, more than 500,000 children with sickle cell disease are born, including 300,000 in Africa, and half of them die before the age of 5 [2]. The World Health Organisation (WHO) estimates that sickle cell disease contributes to the equivalent of 5% of all under-five mortality on the African continent, and up to 16% in certain West African countries (Nigeria and Ghana) [3]. This mortality rate is much higher than that of children with sickle cell disease living in Europe, where more than 90% of them reach adulthood [4].

The lack of reliable data in most countries makes it difficult to estimate the number of people actually affected worldwide. There are no national registers of the disease, even in developed countries that have had neonatal screening programmes for sickle cell disease (SCD) in place for several years (United States, United Kingdom, France). Various estimates have been published, reporting highly variable S allele distribution frequencies depending on the region. At global level, recent estimates indicate that in 2010, 312,302 SS homozygous newborns and 5,476,407 AS heterozygous newborns were born worldwide. 75.5% of SS homozygous newborns were born in sub-Saharan Africa (235,681), 16.9% in the Arab-Indian region (46,826), 4.6% in the Americas (12,802), 3% in Eurasia (7,493) and 0% in South-East Asia. According to these estimates, 50% of the total number of AS or SS infants were born in specific regions of three countries: Nigeria, India and the DRC. The highest frequencies of Hb S (>10%) are found almost exclusively in sub-Saharan Africa [5].

In some parts of this region, sickle cell disease affects up to 2% of newborns. The frequency of the sickle cell trait (i.e. the percentage of healthy carriers who do not have sickle cell disease) is very high. inherited from only one parent) reaches 10 to 40% in equatorial Africa, 1 to 2% on the North African coast and less than 1% in southern Africa. In West African countries (Ghana and Nigeria), the frequency of the sickle cell trait reaches 15 to 30%.

In Uganda, this rate is 45% among the Baambas [3]. In these African countries, mortality among children under 5 with sickle cell disease can be close to 90%, whereas in all low-income countries worldwide, infant mortality (from all causes) has been reduced since 1990-2010. This high mortality rate among sickle-cell patients is thought to be linked to malnutrition, poverty and a lack of screening and vaccination [6].

While mass screening for sickle cell disease in newborns in France, the UK and the USA has become the norm because of its frequency, the usefulness of early diagnosis and its low cost, this is not the case in countries with limited resources. Detection of this disease at birth leaves an interval of two and a half months in which to implement essential therapeutic and preventive measures. This combination of measures significantly reduces morbidity and mortality during the first five years of life [7]. In France, between 1984 and 2019, neonatal screening for sickle cell disease has led to the identification of 9,260 newborns with sickle cell disease (including 586 in 2019) and 180,687 AS heterozygotes. This screening has enabled the early implementation of prophylactic measures for these children, thanks to a structured health and social fabric. Since screening has been organised, a major reduction in mortality and morbidity has been observed in children with sickle cell disease, particularly with regard to invasive infectious complications, anaemia and neurovascular complications [8].In high-resource settings, such as the US, UK and many European countries, universal newborn screening for haemoglobinopathies has clearly reduced infant mortality from sickle cell disease [9,10]. Diagnostic testing for haemoglobinopathies, whether by newborn screening or later in life, involves a number of laboratory methods, including various electrophoresis techniques (gel or capillary), high-performance liquid chromatography (HPLC), mass spectrometry and genetic testing. All these methods require special, often expensive, equipment and highly qualified personnel [11].

The key to combating early mortality in children with sickle cell disease is rapid diagnosis. This makes it possible to educate parents on the best way to care for their affected children, to recognise important danger signs and to prevent complications through the targeted use of vaccines, antibiotics and anti-malarial drugs. Such measures, which could easily be funded by many countries in sub-Saharan Africa (Angola, Kenya), have succeeded in reducing the high early mortality previously seen in other parts of the world (Europe, North America), and there is no reason to suspect that the same should not be true if widely implemented in resource-limited settings. However, to date, sickle cell diagnostic facilities remain poor in many countries in this region, where they are too often restricted to private facilities and beyond the reach of the majority who would benefit from them [12]. Rapid tests have recently become available. They enable a diagnosis to be made in less than 30 minutes, without the need for a laboratory visit [13].
In the absence of curative measures, neonatal screening makes it possible to start preventive treatment for infectious complications and anaemia before the age of three months, and to inform parents about the disease [14].The Sickle SCAN® test is a rapid, qualitative, lateral flow immunochromatographic assay for haemoglobins A, S and C to identify sickle cell disorders [15].

2. Issues

In the DRC, it is estimated that 20 million Congolese (25% to 30% of the population) carry the sickle cell gene and can pass the disease on to their children, and that almost 2% of children are born with sickle cell disease each year in the country [16,17]. This prevalence ranks the country third in the world after Nigeria and India [3]. The DRC has very high mortality and morbidity rates, with 50-75% of deaths occurring before the age of 5 [18]. The available data on the prevalence of sickle cell disease in a population of newborns in Lubumbashi are based on two preliminary surveys conducted in 2021 and 2018. According to these studies, the prevalence of sickle cell trait among these newborns was 18% (including 7.1% with major sickle cell syndrome) and 15.61% (including 3.47% with major sickle cell syndrome) respectively [19,20]. The fight against sickle cell disease faces two major challenges, namely the need to reduce sickle cell births and to consider how to effectively prevent sickle cell complications in order to improve the life expectancy and comfort of people with sickle cell disease. This is why the WHO has recommended a prevention strategy for the African region to reduce the incidence, morbidity and mortality of the disease [21].

In our environment, clinicians are faced with delays in diagnosing sickle cell disease. They have to wait several days (a certain number of samples are required for analysis because of the high cost of reagents, electrical instability with the possibility of altering the samples, and the lengthy time taken to deliver results) or even several months (families' financial difficulties mean they cannot bear the high cost of electrophoresis directly) before obtaining paraclinical results. Not everyone can afford these tests, and they depend on the financial resources of the families concerned. In the meantime, the disease, and even its complications, progress to an advanced stage, sequelae or death. The helpless doctor is forced to witness the suffering of patients and their families, without knowing what appropriate action to take.

Sickle cell anaemia is not a rare disease in our environment, and any practitioner, whatever their speciality, should be able to follow a patient with sickle cell anaemia and show the importance of neonatal screening to the families concerned and their relatives. This shows the need to use a more efficient diagnostic test for our context, limiting the number of patients lost to follow-up and facilitating early management.

This work provides clinicians with a clinical diagnostic and screening tool (Sickle Scan Test). It will enable them to make an immediate diagnosis and undertake rapid, effective and comprehensive treatment at low cost (estimated at the equivalent of $10). In the DRC, this test has only been used in Kindu to assess the prevalence of sickle cell disease in newborns. Before that, there had been no study of its reliability in newborns. This test has not yet been the subject of a study to test its reliability in newborns in the context of the DRC. As the Sickle Scan test is less costly, rapid and less invasive, it would make neonatal screening more acceptable to the Lush population and improve clinical management. This could enable it to be integrated on a large scale into the national health system, thereby reducing prevalence and mortality and improving the quality of life of people with sickle cell disease. The level of knowledge of healthcare professionals caring for patients with sickle cell disease is thought to influence the quality of care, by having a direct impact on morbidity, mortality and the prevalence of sickle cell disease in children.Taking a systems approach, Figure 1 sets out a conceptual framework integrating the determinants of NHW in our environment.

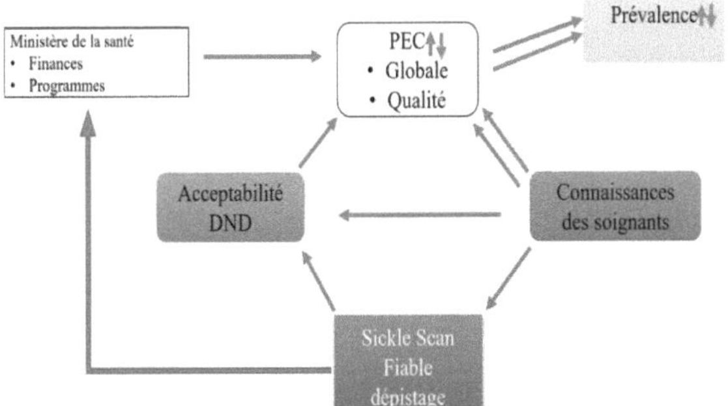

Figure 1: Conceptual framework of the determinants of newborn screening for sickle cell disease

3. Questions for research

Based on our conceptual framework, we believe it would be appropriate to :
• What is the diagnostic reliability of the Sickle scan test in DND in Lubumbashi, which would be an alternative to haemoglobin electrophoresis in our low-resource environment?

• What is the level of acceptability of newborn screening for sickle cell disease and the factors influencing it ;

• What is the prevalence of sickle cell disease among newborns in Lubumbashi?

• What level of knowledge do healthcare providers have about sickle cell anaemia and neonatal screening?

4. Assumptions

The use of sickle cell screening using the Sickle SCAN® test would be feasible and efficient in our environment, with comparable reliability and an alternative to capillary electrophoresis, enabling it to be used systematically and on a large scale in the DRC. The level of acceptability of neonatal screening for sickle cell anaemia by the Lush population would be high and this would give a true prevalence of the disease. The prevalence of sickle cell anaemia in newborns is thought to be higher in Lubumbashi.
The level of knowledge about sickle cell disease and its DND is said to be inadequate among paediatric healthcare staff in Lubumbashi.

5. Objectives

5.1. General objective

The aim of this work is to contribute to improving the survival of children with sickle cell disease in

Through early neonatal diagnosis leading to early treatment.

5.2. Specific objectives

Specifically, the objectives of this work are to :
1. To determine the diagnostic reliability of the Sickle SCAN® test in newborn screening at

Lubumbashi, in reference to Hb electrophoresis.

2. Determine the level of acceptability of NHW and the factors influencing it in the

population of the city of Lubumbashi ;

3. Determining the prevalence of sickle cell disease in newborns in Lubumbashi ;

4. To assess knowledge of sickle cell disease and neonatal screening among healthcare providers in Lubumbashi.

6. Choice and interest of subject

Given the position of the DRC (3ème of countries affected by sickle cell disease), we note that there are no studies on the reliability of the Sickle SCAN® test in neonatal screening for sickle cell disease, the acceptability of neonatal screening for sickle cell disease, or the knowledge of healthcare staff about sickle cell disease. Given the absence of an active national programme for the management of sickle cell anaemia, these studies are a good starting point. starting points in the development of comprehensive, systematic and large-scale care for children with sickle cell disease in the DRC.

References

1. Mattioni S, Stankovic SK, Girota R, Lionneta F. Sickle cell disease in France, revue francophone des laboratoires - april 2016 - n°481// 61-66
2. Pierre A, Bernard AG. Haemoglobinoses tropical diseases Actualités 2022 Updated on 19/04/2022.
3. World Health Organization. Sickle-cell anaemia: Report by the secretariat. Fifty-ninth World Health Assembly A59/9. Item 11.4 of the provisional agenda 24 April 2006
4. Ranque B, Kitenge R, Coulibaly C, Traore H, Adjoumani L, et al. Childhood mortality related to sickle cell disease in sub-Saharan Africa: a multinational study in West and Central Africa. Elsevier ; La Revue de Médecine Interne Volume 42, Supplement 1, June 2021, Page A79.
5. Piel FB, Patil AP, Howes RE, Nyangiri OA, Gething PW, Dewi M, et al. Global epidemiology of sickle haemoglobin in neonates: a contemporary geostatistical model- based map and population estimates. Lancet Lond Engl. 12 Jan 2013;381(9861):142-51.
6. Association for information and prevention of sickle cell disease. Epidemiology 2022. https://apipd.fr/drepanocytose/epidemiologie/ consulted on 01 August 2022
7. Galacteros F. Neonatal diagnosis of haemoglobinopathies. Rev Prat (Paris) 1992; 42(15).

: 1893-1899.

8. Valentine B, Bichr A, Malika B. Neonatal screening for sickle cell disease in France. Médecine/sciences 2021; 37: 482-90
9. Telfer P, Coen P, Chakravorty S, Wilkey O, Evans J, Newell H, Smalling B, Amos R, Stephens A, Rogers D, Kirkham F. Clinical outcomes in children with sickle cell disease living in England: a neonatal cohort in East London. Haematologica. 2007;92:905–912.
10. Quinn CT, Rogers ZR, McCavit TL, Buchanan GR. Improved survival of children and adolescents with sickle cell disease. Blood. 2010;115:3447-3452.
11. Quinn CT, Paniagua MC, DiNello RK, Panchal A, Geisberg M. A rapid, inexpensive and disposable point-of-care blood test for-cell disease using novel, highly specific monoclonal antibodies. Br J Haematol. 2016; 175(4): 724-32.
12. Williams TN. An accurate and affordable test for the rapid diagnosis of sickle cell disease could revolutionize the outlook for affected children born in resource-limited settings. BMC médicine 2015 ; 13 :238.

13. Iserm. Sickle cell anaemia: the most common genetic disease in France 2020. https://www.inserm.fr/dossier/drepanocytose/ 10 November 2022.

14. Orphanet Encyclopaedia for the general public. Sickle Cell Disease. March 2011.

15. Biomedomic. Sickle scan test: instructions for use. BM-SCS-PI-CXJ020-FR.013.

16. Tshilolo L. Sickle cell disease: 10 years of mobilisation against the first genetic disease in the DRC. Https://10 years of mobilisation against the 1st genetic disease in the DRC. Accessed on 26 August 2022.

17. L. Tshiloloa, E. Kafandob, M. Sawadogob, F. Cottonc, F. Vertongenc, A. Fersterd, B. Gulbisc. Neonatal screening and clinical care programmes for sickle cell disorders in sub-Saharan Africa: Lessons from pilot studies. Public Health (2008) 122, 933e941.

18. Plateforme d'appui, de formation et de veille sur la drépanocytose (PAFOVED). Early detection and integrated management of sickle cell disease in the DRC 2012. http://cefacongo.com/updatecefa/files/poster_pafoved/Poster2006%20_2012.pdf

19. Katamea T, Mukuku O, Wembonyama S. Newborn screening for sickle cell disease in Lubumbashi city, Democratic Republic of Congo: a preliminary study on an update of the disease prevalence. BJH 2021; 193 (Suppl. 1): 31

20. Shongo MYP, Mukuku O. Neonatal screening for sickle cell disease in Lubumbashi, DRC.Revue de l'Infirmier Congolais 2018; 2: 62-63.

21. World Health Organization. Sickle cell disease: a strategy for the WHO African Region. Report of the Regional Director 60th session of the Regional Committee for Africa Malabo Equatorial Guinea 30 August - 3 September 2010.

CHAPTER I

GENERAL INFORMATION ON NEONATAL SCREENING FOR SICKLE CELL ANAEMIA

I.1. Newborn screening

I.1.1. Presentation

Neonatal screening is a public health initiative designed to detect certain rare but serious diseases, most of which are genetic in origin, in all newborn babies. The aim is to implement appropriate measures before symptoms appear, in order to avoid or limit the negative consequences of these diseases on children's health [1]. The screening test is not intended to diagnose the disease, but to identify it. If the test is positive, it leads to additional confirmatory examinations, specific to the suspected pathology and capable of establishing a definite diagnosis [2].

The history of systematic newborn screening (NBS), based on dried bloodstains on blotting paper, dates back to 1963 with the development of a test to detect phenylketonuria (PKU), the "Guthrie test", carried out at three days of age. This test measures the amount of phenylalanine (PHE) in the blood and thus its elevation, which is toxic for the child's cerebral development. PKU, a hereditary disease with autosomal recessive transmission, emerged as the first preventable mental retardation thanks to the early establishment of a specific diet low in PHE at a pre-symptomatic stage, enabling children to remain normal. The concept of DNN using blood drops was born. It was introduced in France more than 40 years ago, following Guthrie's discovery, and since then other screening tests using this "Guthrie" blotting paper have been progressively introduced in most developed countries [3].

Currently, 6 diseases are screened at birth [4,5]:

• **Phenylketonuria**: a genetic disease caused by a deficiency in an enzyme that converts the phenylalanine present in food. If left untreated, it can lead to severe mental retardation and neuropsychiatric complications;

• **Congenital hypothyroidism**: a condition in which the thyroid gland does not secrete enough thyroid hormone. I f left untreated, this dysfunction has an impact on the body's major functions and can have a serious impact on the health of the body.

This can lead to severe mental retardation;

• **Congenital adrenal hyperplasia**: a genetic defect in the functioning of the adrenal glands. If left untreated, it can cause severe, sometimes fatal, acute dehydration and impaired development of the sexual organs;

• **Cystic fibrosis**: a genetic disease that leads to severe and repeated respiratory infections and digestive complications;

• **MCAD (Medium-Chain-Acyl-CoA Dehydrogenase) deficiency**: a disease which causes the body to have difficulty using fats as a source of energy. If left untreated, it can lead to coma and even death;

• **Sickle cell anaemia**: a genetic disease linked to the presence of abnormal haemoglobin in the blood, which can lead to persistent anaemia, vascular complications, painful attacks and repeated infections.

• **Galactosemia**: a genetic disease caused by a deficiency in galactose kinase, characterised by an increase in the plasma concentration of galactose and resulting in digestive, neurological, metabolic and growth disorders.

DNN therefore consists of identifying, from among all newborns, those who are likely to have a disease and who, by benefiting from early diagnosis, will have access to effective treatment capable of modifying the course of their disease before irreversible lesions appear [3].

I.1.2. Criteria for screening

For a disease to benefit from a systematic screening programme for all newborns, it must theoretically meet the ten World Health Organisation criteria defined by Wilson and Jungner in 1968 [6].

Screening must therefore :
1° Concern a disease which is a major public health problem; 2° Be accepted by the population;
3° concern a known and well understood disease; 4° be carried out at a pre-symptomatic stage;

5° Be validated by specific tests;

6° Be carried out by a reliable method that has few false positives and few false negatives;
7° Be accompanied by a precise therapeutic protocol; 8° Lead to effective treatment;
9° Be cost-effective; 10° Be sustainable.

1.1.3. Method direct debit

In most countries, a newborn blood sample is required for screening tests [7]. The sample should be taken no earlier than 48 hours after birth, and no later than 72 hours. [8].
Newborn heel puncture to obtain capillary blood has been one of the factors contributing to the success of systematic neonatal screening, due to its simplicity and high rate of technical success by carers. However, for several years now, a good number of centres have been collecting blood from venipunctures, by choice and for some children out of necessity. The main reason given for this choice is to reduce pain, either because venipuncture is less painful than heel pricking, or to reduce the number of injections [9].

I.2. Newborn screening for sickle cell disease

I.2.1. Interest

The aim is to put in place specialised care from birth and measures to prevent infectious complications for children with sickle cell disease (daily antibiotic prophylaxis and special attention to vaccinations), as well as measures to support parents (information on early clinical signs, how the disease is transmitted, what to do in the event of fever or painful attacks, what to do in an emergency, and raising awareness of the importance of close monitoring), how the disease is transmitted, what to do in the event of fever or painful attacks, what to do in an emergency, and the importance of close monitoring), before the first symptoms appear. Subsequent management involves multiple acute and chronic complications linked to anaemia and vaso-occlusive phenomena [10].

Sickle cell disease is associated with significant morbidity and mortality in young children. In 1986, it was shown that prophylactic penicillin therapy reduced the risk of pneumococcal sepsis in patients with sickle cell disease. As a result, a number of neonatal screening policies were rapidly introduced [11].
In the USA, the average annual mortality rate linked to sickle cell disease in children under the age of 5 fell from 2.05 per 100,000 between 1979 and 1989 to 0.47 per 100,000 between 2015 and 2017. [12]; whereas before the 1970s, very few children survived beyond the age of 10 [13]. In France, too, life expectancy for people with sickle cell disease has improved considerably, and the median age at death doubled between 1979-1986 and 2003-2010 [14]. According to the WHO, the situation in Africa shows that current national policies and plans are inadequate, that appropriate facilities and trained personnel are rare, and that diagnostic tools and appropriate treatments are insufficient [15].

I.2.2. Benefits of neonatal screening for sickle cell disease

Although there is no randomised study evaluating the benefit of neonatal screening for sickle cell disease, numerous observational studies have demonstrated the positive impact of this on the prognosis of the disease [16]. Combined with an organised health and social network, neonatal screening for this disease makes it possible to introduce prophylactic measures at an early stage and to help parents recognise the symptoms of clinical complications so that they can seek urgent medical attention if necessary [17].
Survival at 5 years in sickle cell patients, an indicator of early mortality from septicaemia, also appears to have increased: 96.8% (1983-1990), 97.5% (1991-2000) and 99.2% (2001-2007) and at 18 years 93.9%. [18]. Currently in France, the incidence rate of deaths from all causes in children with sickle cell disease is low overall, as are deaths related to the disease. [19]. Early detection of the disease means that treatment can be intensified before irreversible organ damage occurs. It is recommended that hydroxyurea treatment be offered to children from the age of 9 months, including those who are asymptomatic. This treatment leads to improvements in laboratory parameters such as total haemoglobin and foetal haemoglobin levels and a reduction in the number of acute clinical events associated with sickle cell disease such as pain and acute chest syndrome (ACS). [20].

I.2.3. Selective screening versus universal screening

Currently in France, newborn screening for sickle cell anaemia is systematic for all newborns in the overseas departments, regions and collectivities, whereas it is targeted in mainland France. Targeting concerns newborns whose parents belong to a group at risk of sickle cell anaemia. When it is based on geographical origin, it is regularly called into question because of the difficulty of identifying subjects at risk: imprecise answers from couples questioned about their geographical origins, intermingling of populations, medically-assisted procreation, adoptions, etc. Generalising neonatal screening for sickle cell disease would simplify the process, limiting the feeling of stigmatisation and facilitating recognition of sickle cell disease as a public health problem [21].

A recent study carried out between February and May 2017 in the Paris region showed that targeted screening was inadequate. In fact, 5 cases (7.5%) of newborns with major sickle cell syndrome and 155 newborns with AS/AC trait were diagnosed, even though they were considered off-target [22].

I.2.4. Announcement diagnostic

A consultation to announce the diagnosis of a major sickle cell syndrome requires an expert practitioner, or team of practitioners. It generally takes place in two phases, with two consultations staggered over time. The aim is to tell a family about a chronic, potentially severe genetic disease that can affect the whole family, while at the same time including the child in a life project. This is a founding moment in the relationship between doctor and patient, very often sealing a therapeutic alliance that will condition the future [17]. In practice, during the first consultation, the very strong suspicion of sickle cell anaemia is announced. This is an opportunity to ask the parents about their knowledge of the disease and their perception of it. The pathophysiological basis of the disease is explained. After a full clinical examination, the child undergoes biological confirmation based on a haemoglobin study, systematically supplemented by a haemogram, with measurement of the number of reticulocytes, and an iron profile, in order to rule out any deficiency likely to influence haematological parameters. A test for glucose-6-phosphate dehydrogenase (G6PD) deficiency, the enzyme that enables red blood cells to withstand stress. oxidative damage, is generally combined with this initial work-up, given its high prevalence in populations at risk of sickle cell disease and in order to implement the necessary preventive measures at an early stage. Finally, a request for blood group determination with an extended phenotype is made, in order to identify at an early stage a rare blood group associated with sickle cell disease [23].A second consultation, ideally within a month of the first, will enable the diagnosis to be confirmed and preventive treatment to be started (antibiotic prophylaxis with oral penicillin taken twice daily and folate supplementation). This consultation will also provide an opportunity to ensure that the signs of surveillance are properly understood and to answer any questions raised by the diagnosis. Therapeutic education sessions may be offered [17].

I.3. Diagnosis of sickle cell anaemia

There are three main groups of methods [24] :

o The haematological approach with the establishment of the blood-formula count

(CBC) and smear study;

o The haemoglobin study itself, with demonstration of the abnormality phenotypic ;

o The genetic approach, with identification of the mutation directly or indirectly responsible for the phenotypic abnormalities.

I.3.1. Approach haematology

The result of the CBC is essential for interpreting the results of a study of haemoglobin, especially in haemoglobinopathies.Reticulocytes are frequently elevated because the anaemia is regenerative, although erythropoiesis is not very effective. Medullary biopsy is rarely necessary.

I.3.2. Study of haemoglobins

It is based on the detection of differences in electrophoretic mobility or retention time in a chromatography column. It should be remembered that haemoglobins are amphoteric proteins rich in basic amino acids (Arg, Lys) and acidic amino acids (Glu, Asp), with isoelectric points (pI) close to 7. The mutations will affect the amino acids with different charges leading to differences in separation by electrophoretic or chromatographic methods, with modification of the pI giving forms observable by isoelectrofocusing.

The limitations of these separative methods are intrinsically those of the sometimes minimal differences in charge; there are also difficulties in quantification, especially with electrophoretic methods on gels; finally, automation is limited, even though automated chromatography or capillary electrophoresis systems have greatly improved the management of these diseases.

I.3.2.1. Electrophoretic methods on gels

For a long time, electrophoresis (EP) on cellulose acetate gel and then agarose gel was used under alkaline conditions (alkaline EP) in parallel with another electrophoresis carried out under acidic conditions (acid EP). Another approach is the use of gel-based isoelectrofocusing (IEF). Now, all these methods are applicable to capillary electrophoresis (CE), zone electrophoresis (CZE) or capillary isoelectrofocusing (CIEF).

a. In alkaline EP, haemoglobins are negatively charged because the pH (8 to 9) is higher than that of Hb S (6.75 to 7.5). Currently, high-resolution (HR) agarose gels, pH 8.6 buffers and amidoschwarz staining of the gels are used. All haemoglobins will migrate from the cathode, where they have been deposited, towards the anode (anodic migration); they are slowed down by the electroendosmosis flow and migrate at a speed in reverse order to the pi. Hb A is the fastest (pI = 6.98), followed by Hb F (pI = 7.05) then Hb S and Hb D (pI $\approx$ 7.20), and finally Hb A2 (pI = 7.42) which migrates like many abnormal Hb (Hb C, Hb E, Hb O- Arab...).

However, we cannot be certain of the identity of Hb S because other variants, including those in group D such as Hb D-Punjab, which is common in India, can migrate to the same level. All Hb S variants, even sickle cell traits, need to be verified by another method, such as acid EP.

b. Acid PE provides a diagnosis of certainty (or almost!). In this case, the haemoglobins are positively charged because the pH of the citrate buffer (6.2) is lower than that of the acid buffer.

pI of HbS. All haemoglobins will migrate from the anode, where they were deposited, to the cathode (cathodic migration). They migrate in pi order, or thereabouts. In agarose gel/citrate buffer, Hb C migrates towards the anode, carried away by the flow of electroendosmosis, Hb S migrates very little, Hb A is faster but migrates in a group also containing Hb A2, Hb D and Hb E. Hb F is the fastest, along with Hb A1c.

Thus, Hb S that migrate together in alkaline EP (S and D, on the one hand; C and E, on the other hand) are more likely to be present in the blood. part), migrate differently in acid EP (S is separated from D, and C is separated from E).

c. Isoelectrofocusing is another alternative to the previous two. It goes back a long way and is still the benchmark. The principle is very simple. The Hb S will migrate in a pH gradient established in a gel with Ampholines© (a mixture of amino acids of different pI). Each Hb will stop (it is said to 'focus') at a pH value equal to its intrinsic pI, because at this value the amphoteric protein is no longer charged (neutral zwiterrion form, with as many positive as negative charges). Hb S with different pi will be found at different positions in the pH gradient, Hb S that can be identified using controls deposited in parallel. We use polyacrylamide or HR agarose gels, Ampholines© and more rarely Immobilines© (ampholines immobilised on the gel) chosen to form a pH gradient between 6 and 9. The gradient is established at the same time as electrical focusing.

I.3.2.2. Capillary electrophoresis methods

They have now taken on a major role with the development of automated systems that also perform serum protein electrophoresis, CDT (Carbohydrate Desialylated Transferrin) and HbA1c. The quantification of minor fractions (Hb A1c, Hb A2, Hb F, ...) is easy and as good as in chromatography, at least in principle by estimating the area under the peak. The electrophoregram takes about 20 minutes to complete. Quantification is easy and the resolution high. Separation methods are varied.Electrophoretic methods, and in particular IEF and capillary electrophoresis, are very effective and remain essential. However, it is important to be aware that they cannot identify all the variants, on the one hand structural variants whose pI are very close to the most common variants, and on the other hand structural variants affecting the binding of haem without modifying the solubility of Hb (these variants are methemoglobinising : $Fe2+ \rightarrow Fe\ 3+$), and non-structural variants which reduce the affinity of Hb for O2 (e.g. Hb-Hope due to the $\beta36Glu \rightarrow Asp$ mutation) without affecting its solubility or even its stability.

I.3.2.3. Chromatographic methods [25,26]

Chromatography is a chemical analysis technique used to separate the constituents of a mixture. It is an alternative, and in fact a complement, to electrophoretic methods.

The principle of chromatography is based on the differences in affinity of the compounds in a mixture between a mobile phase and a stationary phase. More precisely, the different constituents of the mixture are carried along by the mobile phase and are gradually separated on the fixed (or stationary) phase according to their adsorption or solubility ($\rightarrow$ solution), depending on the chromatographic technique used.

The mobile phase can be either a liquid (in which case it is called the eluent) or a gas (in which case it is called the carrier gas).

The fixed phase can be solid (silica gel, alumina, etc.) or liquid. Each component of the mixture is studied at a characteristic migration speed, which enables it to be separated from the others and thus identified. Generally speaking, the sample is analysed by comparison with substances already known in the sample. The diagram obtained by chromatography is called a chromatogram and shows the variation of the compound studied (minority species) in the mobile phase (eluent or carrier gas) as a function of time. Chromatographic techniques fall into two main categories: liquid chromatography and gas chromatography.

a. Liquid phase chromatography (LPC)

There are different types of liquid chromatography, depending on the separation method used.

• Adsorption chromatography

As its name suggests, this chromatography is based on the selective adsorption of liquid constituents onto the solid phase of the column. In fact, there is a succession of adsorptions and desorptions, the latter being caused by the addition of a solvent at the end of the separation.

• Liquid-liquid partition chromatography

This chromatographic technique uses the difference in solubility ($\rightarrow$ solution) of the constituents in relation to two immiscible liquids.

• Gel permeation or exclusion chromatography (GPC)

Exclusion chromatography uses the difference in penetration of constituents on a polymer gel. As they pass through the column, only molecules whose diameter is less than a certain value can penetrate the pores of the gel. Compounds are thus separated according to the size of their molecules.

• Ion exchange chromatography

This chromatographic technique uses ion exchange between the fixed phase (resin made up of ions) and the mobile phase, which has been ionised beforehand. The ions are generally acids, bases or metal cations. Ion exchange chromatography is used for ionisable substances, particularly in inorganic chemistry.

• Chromatography on paper

In paper chromatography, the mixture to be analysed is first dissolved. A drop of this liquid mixture is placed on a sheet of paper. The solvent migrates by capillary action, carrying with it the various constituents of the mixture, which stop more or less far from the spot formed by the initial drop, depending on their interaction with the cellulose of the paper.

The latter is also used in immunodiagnostics under the name of immunochromataography, which is one of the most modern immunodiagnostic techniques, the main advantages of which are the simplicity and speed of the test.

It can be performed by a simple device developed to detect the presence (or absence) of a target compound in the sample (the matrix). This type of test is commonly used for medical diagnosis, either at home or in the laboratory. It takes the form of a strip in which the sample under test migrates along a solid substrate by capillary action.

Immunochromataography is based on the migration of a sample through a nitrocellulose membrane. The sample is added to the starting zone containing a conjugated detection reagent, which consists of a specific antibody against one of the epitopes of the antigen to be detected and a detection reagent.

In principle, any coloured particle can be used as a detection reagent, but latex (blue in colour) or nano-sized gold particles (red in colour) are the most commonly used.

If the sample contains the target antigen, it binds to the conjugate reagent forming an immune complex and migrates with it along the nitrocellulose membrane. Otherwise, the conjugate reagent and sample will migrate separately without binding.

The capture zone is formed by a second antibody specific for another epitope of the antigen. When the sample reaches this zone, the complexes formed by the binding of the antigen and the conjugate are retained and the line is coloured red or blue (positive samples). Otherwise, the samples are negative.

Most tests include a second line which contains another antibody (not specific to the assay) that binds to some of the remaining coloured particles that did not bind to the control line. This confirms that the liquid has passed from the sample application pad to the test line. By confirming that the sample has had the opportunity to interact with the test line, it increases confidence that a visibly altered test line can be interpreted as a negative result.

- **High performance liquid chromatography (HPLC)**

This technique has become one of the most widely used in chemical analysis laboratories, thanks to its extreme precision, which enables trace compounds to be detected. Coupled with an appropriate detection method, forced-flow chromatography enables a wide variety of organic or inorganic compounds to be identified and quantified.

b. Gas chromatography (GC)

Gas chromatography is used to separate mixtures of gases or compounds that can be vaporised at high temperature. The mixture to be analysed is injected into a metal column a few millimetres in diameter containing the fixed phase. The compounds are carried under pressure by a gas (known as the carrier gas). This is generally helium (He), argon (Ar) or nitrogen (N2).

I.3.2.4. Other biochemical methods [27] :

• The Emmel test, which consists of placing a drop of blood on a slide in the presence of a drop of 2% sodium metabisulphite. The slide is lined with paraffin.

Examination under the microscope after 30 minutes shows a sickle-shaped appearance of the red blood cells,

• The Itano test is a haemoglobin solubility test performed on haemoglobin haemolysate adjusted to 4%. In the presence of sodium hyposulphite, haemoglobin S precipitates. After centrifugation, a pink clot and a clear supernatant are observed in the presence of Hb S; in the absence of Hb S, the supernatant is red.

I.3.3. Genetic study [24]

It is of interest in 3 cases:

• Phenotypic data are insufficient to establish a diagnosis (especially for β-thalassemias);
• Prenatal diagnosis of sickle cell disease ;

• Prenatal diagnosis of α-thalassaemia type 4 and β-thalassaemia major, with knowledge of the mutation or deletion in the parents.
The results are not always successful, and phenotype/genotype correlations are not always good. The techniques used include reverse dot blot, classical or multiplex PCR, digital PCR, Sanger sequencing and NGS (new generation sequencing).

References

1. French National Authority for Health (HAS). Newborn screening: which diseases to screen for? Press release - online 03 Feb 2020. https://www.has-sante.fr/jcms/p_3149627/en/depistage-neonatal-quelles-maladies-depister Accessed 29 Aug 2022.
2. Samuel Amintas. Stability study of neonatal screening markers on dried blood spots on blotting paper. Pharmaceutical Sciences. 2018. ffdumas-01876510. https://dumas.ccsd.cnrs.fr/dumas-01876510/document
3. Roussey M. Le dépistage néonatal. 2010-2011. http://campus.cerimes.fr/genetique-medicale/enseignement/genetique13/site/html/cours.pdf Accessed 29 August 2022.
4. French National Authority for Health (HAS). Neonatal screening: The HAS plays an active role in the national programme articlehas -mis online at online on 18 Nov. 2021. https://www.has- sante.fr/jcms/p_3296719/en/depistage-neonatal-la-has-partie-prenante-du-programme- national Accessed 29 August 2022.
5. Succoio M, Sacchettini R, Rossi A, Parenti G, et al. Galactosemia: Biochemistry, Molecular Genetics, Newborn Screening, and Treatment. Biomolecules 2022, 12, 968. https://doi.org/10.3390/biom12070968
6. Wilson J and Jungner Y. Principles and practice of screening for disease 1968. Geneva, WHO: 26-39
7. Vibhuti S and Arne O. Venepuncture versus heel lance for blood sampling in term neonates 05 October 2011. https://doi.org/10.1002/14651858.CD001452.pub4. Accessed August 30, 2022.
8. PACA-Corsica Regional Neonatal Screening Centre. Neonatal screening programme. 1 December 2020.
9. Carbajal R, Gatterre P, Rambaud J and De Suremain N. Pain and newborn screening. Archives de pédiatrie, 2016/03,Vol 23 (N° 3), pages 229-231, 17 ref.
10. French National Authority for Health (HAS). Newborn screening for sickle cell disease in France. 11 March 2014.
11. Zentech SA. Rare diseases haemoglobinopathies (sickle cell disease) 2018.

12. Amanda BP, Jason MM, Christina C, Dana LH, Lisa CR, Christopher JB, W Craig H. Trends in Sickle Cell Disease-Related Mortality in the United States, 1979 to 2017. Ann

Emerg Med. 2020;76:S28-S36.

13. Chakravorty S, Williams TN. Sickle cell disease: a neglected chronic disease of increasing global health importance. Arch Dis Child 2015; 100:48-53. doi :10.1136/archdischild- 2013-303773.
14. Gomes E, Castetbon K, Goulet V. Sickle cell disease mortality in France: age of death and associated causes (1979-2010). 10 March 2015
15. World Health Organization. Sickle cell disease: a strategy for the WHO African Region. Report by the Regional Director. Sixtieth session Malabo, Equatorial Guinea, 30 August - 3 September 2010.
16. Lees C, Davies SC, Dezateux C. Neonatal screening for sickle cell disease. Cochrane Database Syst Rev 2000. doi.org/10.1002/14651858.CD001913.
17. Valentine B, Bichr A, Malika B. Neonatal screening for sickle cell disease in France. 18 May 2021. https://hal.archives-ouvertes.fr/hal-03229323 consulted on 31 August 2022.
18. Quinn CT, Rogers ZR, Mccavit TL, et al. Improving survival of children and adolescents with sickle cell disease. Blood. 2010 ; 115 (17) :3447-52.
19. Desselas E, Thuret I, Kaguelidou F, et al. Mortality in children with sickle cell disease in mainland France from 2000 to 2015. Hematological 2020; 105: e440-3. 19
20. Yawn BP, Buchanan GR, Afenyi-Annan AN, et al. Management of sickle cell disease: summary of the 2014 evidence-based report by expert panel members. JAMA 2014; 312: 1033-48.

21. Bichr A, Nathalie C, Mariane DM. Neonatal screening for sickle cell disease and pathways d'organisation des soins. La Revue du Praticien. Published on 20 April 2019; 69(4) ;411

22. Cavazzana M, Stanislas A, Rémus C, et al. Neonatal screening for sickle cell disease: data in favour of its generalisation. Med Sci (Paris) 2018; 34: 309-11.

23. Haute Autorité de Santé. Management of sickle cell disease in children and adolescents.Paris: HAS, 2005.

24. Bruno B. Haemoglobin diseases: normal and pathological haemoglobins. Revue francophone des laboratoires - april 2016 - n°481 : 27-33
25. https://www.larousse.fr/encyclopedie/divers/chromatographie/33792. Retrieved from on14

February 2022

26. https://fr.wikipedia.org/wiki/Immunochromatographie Accessed on 15 February 2022

27. Pierre A, Bernard AG. Haemoglobinoses tropical diseases Actualités 2022 Updated on 19/04/2022.

CHAPTER II

METHODOLOGY

II.1.Description of the working environment

II.1.1. Geographical data

Lubumbashi, capital of Haut Katanga Province in the southern part of the country, is the Democratic Republic of Congo's second-largest city in terms of population and its economic capital [1]. It lies between longitudes 27°15′ and 27°40′ East and latitudes 11°26′-11°55′ South. The town was founded around 1906-1910, when copper deposits were discovered and mined by Union Minière du Haut Katanga (U.M.H.K). The company was established on the Lubumbashi site, named after the river that flows through it. It is divided into seven communes (Annexe, Kamalondo, Kampemba, Katuba, Kenya, Lubumbashi and Ruashi) [2].

It has a tropical climate with two seasons. The rainy season is humid and overcast, while the dry season is generally clear. The climate is warm throughout the year, with temperatures generally ranging from 9°C to 34°C, and rarely below 7°C or above 36°C.

• The very hot season lasts 1.9 months, from 10 September to 6 November, with an average daily maximum temperature of over 32°C. The hottest month of the year in Lubumbashi is October, with an average maximum temperature of 34°C and a minimum of 18°C.
• The cool season lasts 7.3 months, from 18 December to 27 July, with an average daily maximum temperature below 27°C. The coldest month of the year in Lubumbashi is June, with an average minimum temperature of 10°C and a maximum of 25°C. [3]

The hydrography is made up of 7 main rivers: Kafubu, Kampemba, Karavia, Lubumbashi, Luano, Naviundu and Ruashi. The vegetation is of the wooded savannah type throughout the periphery, with a few forest galleries in the north [4].

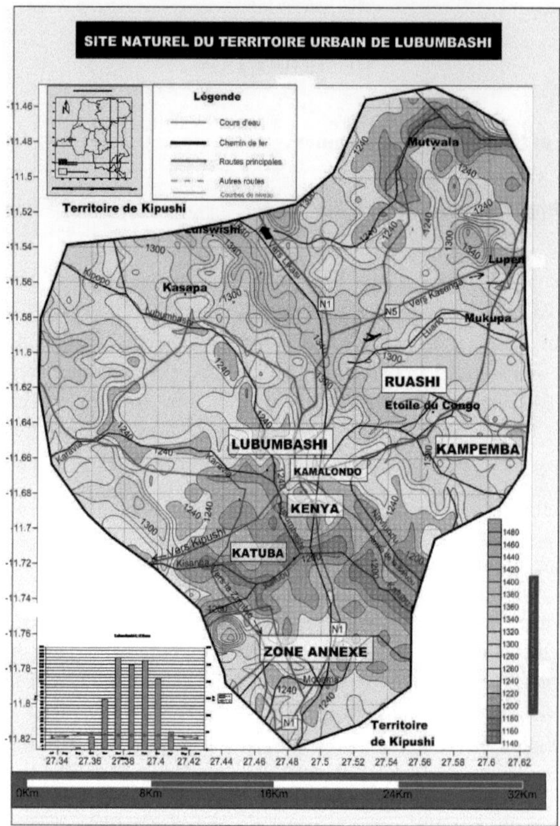

Figure 2. Natural site in the urban area of Lubumbashi, (RDCMAPS on 29-11-2010) [4].

II.1.2. Population and activities

The population of Lubumbashi is heterogeneous and estimated at 2,478,262 in 2020 over an area of 900 km^2 [5]. The city of Lubumbashi is a major commercial centre and mining zone, where several indigenous tribes and other tribes from the DRC and Africa live side by side. A diversity of traditional values constitutes a rich cultural and artistic potential for the city of Lubumbashi. Almost 50% of the population survives mainly through small-scale trade. As Lubumbashi is essentially a mining town, around 25% of the population work in the mining industries [1,6].

II.1.3. Lubumbashi health zones

The city of Lubumbashi has 251 health facilities (219 primary care facilities, 23 intermediate care facilities and 9 hospitals) spread across 11 health zones (ZS) located in different commues of the city: ZS Lubumbashi, ZS Kampemba, ZS Katuba, ZS Kenya, ZS Kisanga, ZS Kowe, ZS Kamalondo, ZS Mumbunda, ZS Ruashi, ZS Tshamilemba and ZS Vangu. With the exception of the ZS Kowe (Special Health Zone of the Congolese National Police), each general referral hospital offers complementary activities. Maternity wards are available in almost 2/3 of front-line facilities, in all intermediate facilities and in all hospitals. Nine out of ten births are assisted [7].

Lubumbashi also has a provincial general referral hospital (Hôpital Jason Sendwe) and a university clinic (Cliniques Universitaires de Lubumbashi). These two facilities receive patients from several localities, regions and general referral hospitals, and currently have a university vocation (teaching, training and research). These two health facilities (FOSA) serve as a reference for all the other facilities in the Haut Katanga Province health system, particularly in terms of neonatal care.

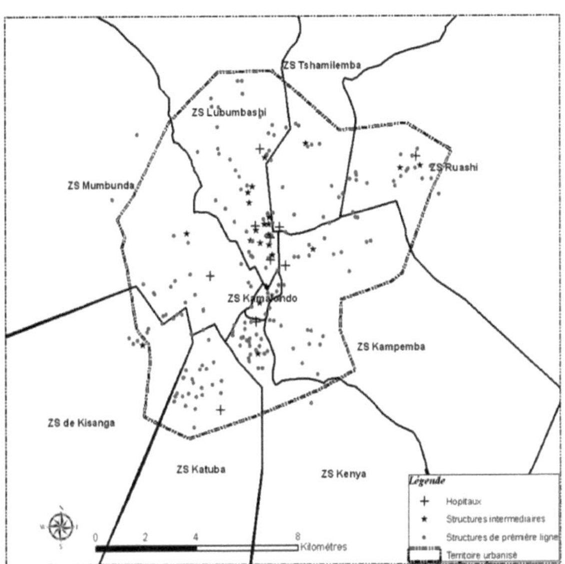

Figure 3: Spatial location of health care facilities in Lubumbashi in 2006 [7].

II.2. Types of study

In the present work, the studies will be defined by objective set according to the analysis framework.

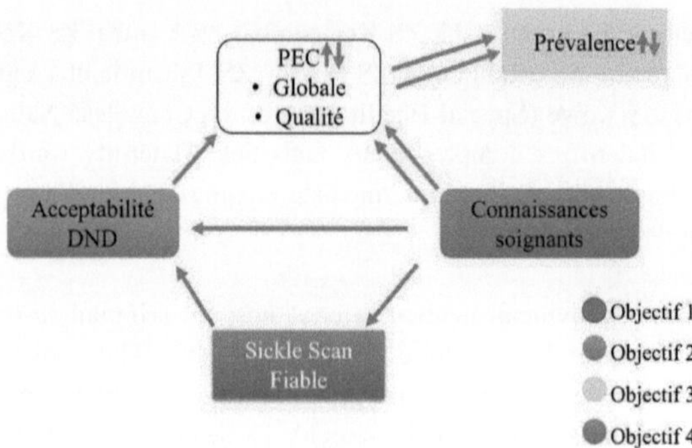

Figure 4: Analysis framework based on objectives

Table I. Summary of objectives and types of study carried out

Objectifs	Type d'étude	Population	Période	Echantillon	Cadre d'étude
Déterminer la fiabilité diagnostique du test rapide Sickle SCAN® dans le DND en référence à l'électrophorèse	Descriptive transversale	Nouveau-nés d'au plus 6 jours	Juin à décembre 2020	365	9 maternités
Déterminer le niveau d'acceptabilité du DND et les facteurs l'influençant	Descriptive transversale à visée analytique	Population Lushoise	Décembre 2020	2032	7 communes
Déterminer la prévalence de la drépanocytaire à Lubumbashi, RDC	Descriptive transversale	Nouveau-nés d'au plus 6 jours	Juin à décembre 2020	538	9 maternités
Evaluer les connaissances des professionnels de santé sur la drépanocytose et son dépistage néonatal	Descriptive transversale à visée analytique	Médecins et infirmiers	Décembre 2020	465	16 FOSA

Objective 1: To determine the diagnostic reliability of the Sickle SCAN® rapid test in neonatal screening for sickle cell disease with reference to haemoglobin electrophoresis in Lubumbashi, Democratic Republic of Congo.

This is a descriptive cross-sectional study comparing the results of the Sickle Scan rapid test and haemoglobin electrophoresis. The study period ran from June to December 2020. It was carried out on 365 newborns aged 6 days or less in 9 maternity units in the city of Lubumbashi, namely the Jason Sendwe General Referral Hospital, the Katuba General Referral Hospital, the Kamalondo General Referral Hospital, the Kenya General Referral

Hospital, the Kisanga Health Zone Hospital, the Ruashi Military Hospital, the Camp Vangu Military Hospital and the Saint François Hospital, as well as at the Lubumbashi University Clinics.

We took two samples: the Sickle SCAN® rapid test, which is an immunochromatographic assay for the qualitative detection of haemoglobins A, S and C, immediately took 5 μl of venous blood from the back of the hand. 500 μl of blood taken from the same site was then conditioned in a cool box at 5° C and flown to the laboratory at Monkole Hospital in Kinshasa (DRC) for capillary electrophoresis (carried out using a new-generation machine, the Capillarys 2 Flex Piercing System [Sebia SA, France]). Training was provided for research assistants and nurse advisers. Pre-test counselling was carried out for all consenting mothers. The duration of the education was approximately 30 minutes and depended on the mothers' questions. Post-test counselling was carried out the same day after the results of the Sickle scan test, while the results of the confirmatory test were communicated by telephone within 10 days. Children who tested positive for sickle cell disease were referred to our principal investigator for follow-up and medical management.

Sickle Scan test analysis procedure :

✓ 5μl of venous blood on the back of the newborn's hand using a micropipette.
✓ Injection of the sample into the buffer solution (1ml)
✓ 5 drops of the treated sample solution are placed in the collection well of the cartridge.

✓ Read the results after 5 minutes.

✓ A total of four detection lines can be present in this procedure: HbA, HbS, HbC and control line.

The Sickle Scan Kit consists of a 5 μl micropipette, a buffer solution and a cassette. The data was entered into Excel 2019 and analysed using STATA software (version 16).

Objective 2: To assess the acceptability of neonatal screening for sickle cell disease and the factors influencing it in Lubumbashi in the Democratic Republic of Congo.

The aim of this study was to determine the level of acceptability of NHW and the factors influencing it in Lubumbashi using a descriptive cross-sectional method with an analytical focus. It was carried out in December 2020. It was carried out on a population from the various communes of the city of Lubumbashi, with a minimum age of 18. 2032 participants were selected. The closed, self-administered and contextualised Wonkam questionnaire was used for the survey. This questionnaire was designed to collect information from respondents on socio-demographic characteristics, knowledge of DND, attitudes towards sickle cell screening policies and attitudes towards voluntary termination of pregnancy if the participant's unborn child were to be affected by sickle cell disease. A pilot study of ten selected participants was conducted to determine whether the questionnaire items were easy to understand. The pilot interviews were used to ensure that no ambiguous questions were asked and to determine the time required to complete an interview. The surveys lasted an average of 25 minutes. The data obtained during the pilot interviews were not included in the final results of this study. Three teams, each consisting of six interviewers, were formed to collect the data. The survey form was either completed by the interviewer if the person could not read or write, or completed by the respondent after clarification by the interviewer. The team received training over three days before and after the pre-test. This covered interview techniques, the purpose of the study and ethical aspects. The principal investigator and supervisors monitored the site on a daily basis throughout the data collection period and checked that each questionnaire was fully completed in order to ensure its completeness and consistency. The data was entered into Excel 2019 and analysed using STATA software (version 15).

Objective 3: To determine the prevalence of sickle cell disease in Lubumbashi, Democratic Republic of Congo.

The main objective of this descriptive cross-sectional study was to calculate the prevalence of sickle cell disease in newborns in Lubumbashi. It was carried out on 538 newborns aged 6 days or less in 9 maternity units in the city of Lubumbashi, namely the Jason Sendwe Provincial General Reference Hospital, the Katuba General Reference Hospital, the Kamalondo General Reference Hospital, the Kenya General Reference Hospital, the Kisanga Health Zone Hospital, the Ruashi Military Hospital, the Camp Vangu Military Hospital and the Saint François Hospital, as well as the Lubumbashi University Clinics, during the period from June to December 2020. A maximum of 500 µl of blood sample was taken in microtainer tubes of ethylene diamine tetra acetic acid (EDTA) from the venipuncture of the back of the hand of each newborn in the selected health facilities. The newborn blood samples were then conditioned in a cool box at 5° C and flown to the laboratory at Monkole Hospital in Kinshasa (DRC), where capillary electrophoresis (using a new-generation machine, the Capillarys 2 Flex Piercing System [Sebia SA, France]) was carried out. Research assistants and nurse advisers were trained. Pre-test counselling was carried out for all consenting mothers.Health education was provided prior to obtaining consent for a newborn to be screened. The duration of the education was approximately 30 minutes and depended on the mothers' questions. Health education on sickle cell disease was provided through a short interview with a group of mothers. The information included the origin of sickle cell disease, the different types of sickle cell status, the importance of clinic visits and healthy lifestyles. Training was provided in Swahili and/or French to ensure comprehension. The results of the sickle cell screening were communicated to all the mothers, along with post-test counselling. Children who tested positive for sickle cell disease were referred to the paediatrician, the principal investigator, for follow-up and further advice. The data were entered into Excel 2019 and analysed using STATA software (version 16).

Objective 4: To assess healthcare professionals' knowledge of sickle cell disease and neonatal screening in Lubumbashi, Democratic Republic of Congo.

It is also a descriptive cross-sectional study with analytical aims, conducted from 1er to 31 December 2020, to determine the level of knowledge about sickle cell disease and its neonatal screening in Lubumbashi. It focused on healthcare providers working in paediatrics, i.e. 204 doctors and 261 nurses in various medical facilities in the Lubumbashi health district.

Table II. Selection of health facilities

PUBLIC HOSPITALS		PRIVATE FOSA	
Stage 1		STAGE 1	
Comprehensive hospital screening	9 hospitals	Convenience and random sorting	15 CP
Convenience and random sorting of CS	1 CUL 15 CS	CS and CP	15 CS
Stage 2		STAGE 2	
Resonant choice (minimum of	5 hospitals	Resonated choice (minimum of 50	5 CP
50 deliveries/month) Convenience triage and random	1 CS 1 CUL	births/month) Convenience and random sorting	4 CS
Total	7		9

We carried out multi-stage sampling. At the first stage, concerning the public facilities, we carried out an exhaustive sampling of all the hospitals and university clinics in Lubumbashi and we carried out a random selection of the various public (25) and private (30) health facilities (CS and CP). At the second stage, by reasoned choice, we selected 5 health facilities per category (CS, Hospitals, CP) with a minimum of 50 deliveries per month, i.e. 16 health facilities.The health facilities selected for the study are the Light, Yahweh Rafa. CPP, Shaloom, Saint Clément, the general referral hospitals of Kampemba, Katuba, Kenya, Kisanga, Sendwe, the private clinics of Saint François, Holiness, Baume de Galade, Hope, Mane cachée and the university clinics of Lubumbashi. Two contextualised, closed and self-administered questionnaires were used. The Diniz questionnaire was used to assess healthcare professionals' knowledge of sickle cell disease. It consisted of 13 questions, each containing 4 to 6 assertions, of which only one was correct. The score ranged from 0 to 13. Concerning the assessment of knowledge about DND, the Walter's questionnaire of 4 items, each consisting of 2 assertions, was used. Only one assertion was correct. The score ranged from 0 to 4. A pilot study was conducted with 16 health professionals from 2 health facilities (CUL and HPGR Jason Sendwe).

Participants were asked to complete the questionnaires and provide feedback on the relevance, clarity and difficulty of the questionnaire items. Participants expressed no difficulties with the questionnaires and this led to their adoption for the survey itself. The interviewers recruited received training, covering the context of the actual survey, detailed interpretation of the survey instruments and a mock survey test. Finally, a total of 10 interviewers were recruited. The interviewers explained the purpose and procedure of the study and obtained informed consent from each respondent before asking them to complete the questionnaires. On average, the survey lasted between 10 and 15 minutes. The data collected were also entered into Excel 2019 and analysed using STATA software (version 15). The level of knowledge of healthcare professionals about sickle cell disease in general will have an influence on the acceptability of DND by the population, which should make it possible to introduce or activate a large-scale systematic DND programme in our setting.

II.3.Ethical considerations

Our research work obtained prior authorisation from the medical ethics committee of the University of Lubumbashi (approval number UNILU/CEM/030/2021) after submission of the research protocol.Secondly, favourable opinions from the authorities of each health institution enabled us to carry out our field research, after presentation of the research certificates obtained from the Faculty of Medicine of the University of Lubumbashi. Before conducting the interviews, an introductory explanation informed the participants of the purpose and method of the study, after which free and informed consent was obtained. We guaranteed the anonymity of the data collected and all those involved in the research were bound by confidentiality. Participants were free to withdraw from the study at any time. The study was conducted on a not-for-profit basis.

References

1. Lubumbashi https://fr.wikipedia.org/wiki/Lubumbashi

2. Ministry of Energy and Hydraulic Resources. Etude d'impact environnemental et social des infrastructures hydrauliques de la ville de Lubumbashi dans la province du haut- Katanga 2018. https://documents1.worldbank.org/curated/es/511821529553513276/pdf/EIES-Lubumbashi.pdf Accessed on 15 November 2022

3. Weather spark.. Climate and year-round weather averages for Lubumbashi Congo-Kinshasa 2022. https://fr.weatherspark.com/y/94251/M%C3%A9t%C3%A9o-moyenne-%C3%A0- Lubumbashi-Congo-Kinshasa-all-year-round accessed 17 November 2022

4. Donatien Kandolo K. Evolution des éléments du climat en RD Congo. Editions universitaires européennes. Available at: http://rdcmaps.centerblog.net/14-site-naturel- de-la-ville-delubumbashi. Accessed on 14 March 2021

5. World Population Review. Lubumbashi Population 2020.

6. Agency for Special Economic Zones. Fiche technique du Haut-Katanga 2017. https://www.azes-rdc.com/index.php?idart=1207&idrub=169&rubhote= consulted on 25 November 2022

7. Chenge M, Van der vennet J, Porignon D, Luboya NO, Kabyla IB and Criel B. La carte sanitaire de la ville de Lubumbashi, République Démocratique du Congo Partie I : problématique de la couverture sanitaire en milieu urbain congolais (2010). Global Health Promotion; 17(3): 63-74.

CHAPTER III

RESULTS

Objective 1: Determine the diagnostic reliability of the Sickle SCAN® rapid test in DND in Lubumbashi, Democratic Republic of Congo.
Authors: *Tina Katamea, Olivier Mukuku, Oscar N. Luboya, Léon Tshilolo, Stanis O. Wembonyama*
Journal: *British Journal of Haematology*

Original article: 2021; 193 (Suppl. 1): 25

1. Summary

Introduction: Sickle cell disease is a common and potentially fatal haematological disorder. Universal screening and early intervention have contributed significantly to reducing infant mortality in high-resource countries. However, people living in low-resource settings are often only diagnosed in late childhood when they show clinical symptoms. The high cost and complexity of conventional diagnostic methods for sickle cell disease limit its neonatal screening in sub-Saharan Africa and other low-resource regions of the world.

Methods: We evaluated the reliability of the Sickle SCAN® test, a qualitative chromatographic lateral flow immunoassay for haemoglobins A, S and C designed to facilitate rapid diagnosis. Samples from 365 neonates were analysed by this rapid method and compared with results from capillary electrophoresis.

Results: The Sickle SCAN® correctly identified the haemoglobin (Hb) phenotype in 97.26% of cases (95% CI: 95.02% - 98.68%). Sensitivity (97.76% [CI95%: 94.85% - 99.27%]) and specificity (96.48% [CI95%: 91.97% - 98.85%]) for the detection of Hb AA were excellent. For Hb AS, sensitivity (95.83% [CI95% : 90.54% - 98.63%]) and specificity (97.96% [CI95% : 95.30% - 99.33%]) were also excellent. There were no false positive or false negative results for the detection of Hb SS and Hb AC, with sensitivities and specificities equal to 100%.

Conclusion: This study demonstrates the potential usefulness of this rapid test in reducing the overall cost and increasing the accessibility of neonatal screening for sickle cell disease in countries with limited resources.

Key words: Sickle cell disease; Neonatal screening; Newborn; Sickle SCAN® ; Lubumbashi.

2. Introduction

Sickle cell anaemia is an inherited blood disorder, the most common in the world and potentially fatal. It is the most common genetic disease, with around 500,000 births per year [1], two-thirds of which occur in Africa [2]. It is characterised by chronic haemolysis, chronic inflammation, immune deficiency, a heterogeneous clinical phenotype and visceral damage. The pathogenic mechanism in sickle cell disease is mainly due to chronic inflammation associated with oxidative stress [3,4].The WHO estimates that sickle cell disease contributes to the equivalent of 5% of all under-five mortality on the African continent, and up to 16% in certain high-prevalence African countries [5,6]. Recent data from a neonatal screening study in Lubumbashi, for example, indicate a birth prevalence of 12.14% for sickle cell trait (Hb AS) and 3.47% for sickle cell major syndrome (Hb SS) [7]. Estimates suggest that up to 50-90% of children born with sickle cell disease in low-income developing countries in sub-Saharan Africa will die before the age of 5 [8,9].

Under-5 mortality is high in sickle cell patients, associated in particular with the Hb SS phenotype in sub-Saharan Africa [10]. The cornerstone of care management is early diagnosis, ideally neonatal, of sickle cell disease to enable rapid parental education and advice on complications of the disease, vaccination and antibiotic prophylaxis [5,11].

Universal screening and early intervention have made a major contribution to reducing infant mortality in developed countries. Universal screening of newborns in the United States and many other developed countries using highly accurate laboratory methods has enabled early intervention and treatment of sickle cell disease. These have significantly reduced sickle cell infant mortality and contributed to an overall improvement in the quality and length of life of people with sickle cell disease [12,13].In developing countries, sickle cell disease is often diagnosed in late childhood when clinical symptoms first appear. The high cost and complexity (providing results several days after blood sampling) of diagnostic methods conventional methods for sickle cell anaemia limit neonatal screening in sub-Saharan Africa and other low-resource regions of the world [14,15]. These methods are neither rapid nor easy to implement in resource-limited settings, as they require a substantial financial investment with constraints: time, regular replenishment of reagents, availability of electricity, mobilisation of dedicated and trained technicians, transport and storage of biological samples and compliance with strict laboratory standards. They also carry a high risk of loss to follow-up, due to the long delay between sample collection and delivery of results, which could exceed 4 to 6 weeks [16]. Recent tests have emerged as potential alternative tools for the reliable and simple diagnosis of sickle cell disease in developing countries. These include BioMedomics' Sickle SCAN®, a sandwich chromatographic immunoassay approach developed for the qualitative measurement of Hb A, Hb S and Hb C in whole blood samples [17]. This test has demonstrated excellent intrinsic performance in detecting common Hb variants [17-21]. However, no studies have been conducted in the DRC in general and in Lubumbashi in particular. The aim of this study is to evaluate the diagnostic reliability of the Sickle SCAN® test in neonatal screening for sickle cell disease in Lubumbashi, DRC, with reference to the high-performance methods used in our laboratories.

3. Materials and methods

3.1. Study framework

The DRC is the 4th most populous country in Africa, with around 105 million inhabitants. Its population is multi-ethnic and culturally diverse, spread across 26 provinces. A World Bank report stated that the DRC has the third highest number of poor people in the world, and the situation has worsened still further in the wake of the COVID-19 pandemic. According to estimates, 73% of its population, or 60 million people, lived on less than $1.90 a day in 2018 (the level set as the international poverty line). Nearly one person in six living in extreme poverty in sub-Saharan Africa lives in the DRC. The Congolese healthcare system is organised into primary, secondary and tertiary levels. Out-of-pocket expenditure by households remained the main source, accounting for 42% of total healthcare expenditure in 2016 [22]. Public spending on health as a percentage of GDP is lower than the African average sub-Saharan Africa. The city of Lubumbashi, capital of Haut-Katanga Province, is located in the south-eastern geopolitical zone of the DRC and has a cosmopolitan population with a mix of Congolese ethnic groups dominated by the Bemba and Luba ethnic groups. It has an estimated population of 2,478,262 million in 2020, covering an area of 900 km^2 .

The study took place in 9 maternity units in the city of Lubumbashi, including Jason Sendwe General Referral Hospital, Katuba General Referral Hospital, Kamalondo General Referral Hospital, Kenya General Referral Hospital, Kisanga Health Zone Hospital, Ruashi Military Hospital, Camp Vangu Military Hospital and Saint François Hospital, as well as the Cliniques Universitaires de Lubumbashi.

3.2. Study population, design, determination of sample size and selection of participants

The study was a descriptive cross-sectional study conducted from June to December 2020. The study population included clinically healthy newborns aged 6 days or less, weighing between 2000g and 4000g; born in the maternity units of the above-mentioned health facilities in Lubumbashi. Newborns were eligible for screening after obtaining verbal informed consent from their mothers. Trained nurses performed the screening.

Cochran's formula for descriptive studies was used to calculate the sample size (n = z pq/d^{22}) [23], with a 95% confidence interval normal standard deviation (1.96), an estimated sickle cell prevalence of 3.47% [7] and a precision error of 2.5% (0.025). The minimum sample size calculated was 206 participants. Taking into account a 20% non-response rate, a sample size of 248 was calculated, but in the end 365 newborns were recruited for the study (Figure 5).

All neonates whose mothers consented between June and December 2020 were included. We excluded all newborns with a history of blood transfusion since birth and who were clinically unstable.

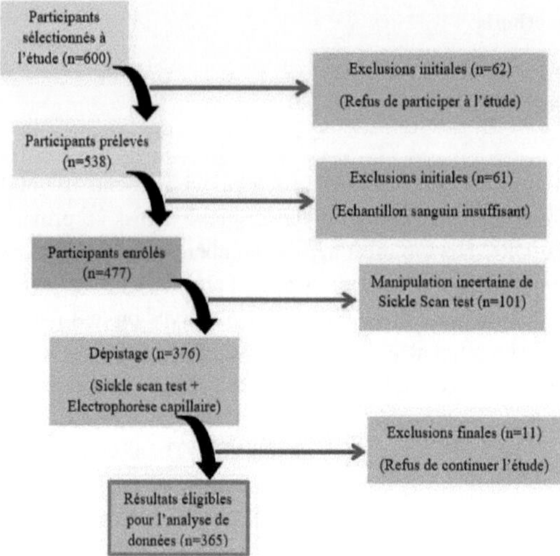

Figure 5. Selection and enrolment of study participants

3.3. Pre-test counselling and participant recruitment

Research assistants and nurse advisors were trained prior to the start of the study. Pre-test counselling was carried out for all consenting mothers by the trained nurse advisers, and informed consent for the test was obtained from the mother of each newborn before the test.

3.4. Blood testing procedures

500 µl of blood were collected by venipuncture from the back of the hand of each of the neonates in an EDTA microtainer tube and 5 µl of blood were collected at the same site for the Sickle SCAN® (BioMedomics, Inc, Morris ville, NC) which is a chromatographic sandwich immunoassay for the qualitative detection of HbA, of human Hb S and Hb C in a blood sample [21]. This is a rapid and reliable test for detecting AA, AS, AC, SS, SC and CC phenotypes [17,21]. It is supplemented by a certainty test which can identify other haemoglobins such as foetal Hb (Hb F) not detected by this rapid screening test.

The Sickle SCAN rapid test® was carried out immediately after the sample was taken. The newborns' blood samples were then packed in a cool box at 5° C and flown to the laboratory at Monkole Hospital in Kinshasa (DRC), where capillary electrophoresis (using a new-generation machine, the Capillarys 2 Flex Piercing System [Sebia SA, France]) was carried out. Sickle SCAN® was compared with capillary electrophoresis as a reference method to determine the accuracy of Sickle SCAN® in detecting Hb AA (normal), AS (HbS trait), AC (Hb C trait), SS (sickle cell anaemia or sickle cell major syndrome), SC (composite heterozygous sickle cell disease) and CC (haemoglobinosis C) phenotypes in the laboratory.

The decision-making algorithm recommended for the detection of haemoglobin S and C, as shown in Figure 6.

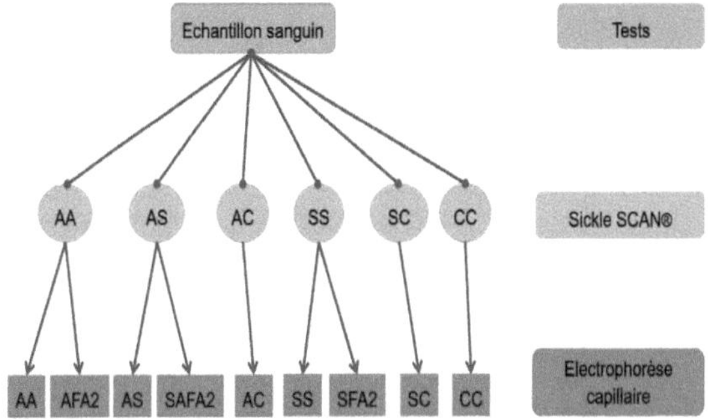

Figure 6. Decision-making algorithm for the diagnosis of sickle cell disease

All Sickle SCAN® tests were performed by the same selected and trained operators in different hospitals chosen for the study. The presence or absence of Sickle SCAN® bands was observed by two different double-blind readers. The Sickle SCAN® phenotype was classified according to the intensity of the Hb band (Figure 7).

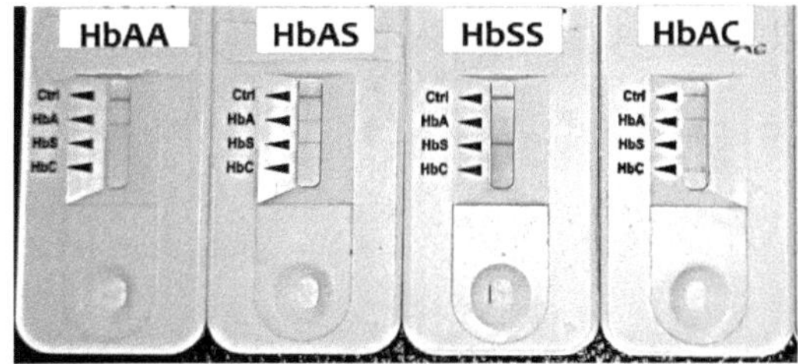

Figure 7: Image showing Sickle SCAN® devices for 4 common haemoglobin profiles seen in our study population.

3.5. Post-test counselling

The results of the Sickle SCAN® test were communicated to all the mothers after a post-test counselling session on the same clinic day, while the results of the confirmatory test were communicated by telephone within 10 days. Children testing positive for sickle cell disease were referred to the principal investigator for follow-up and medical management.

3.6. Statistical analysis

All statistical analyses were performed using STATA 16 (Stata Corp, College Station, TX). For all calculations, the presence or absence of Hb A, Hb S and Hb C detected by the Sickle SCAN® rapid test was compared with the reference result obtained by capillary electrophoresis. Sensitivity, specificity, positive and negative predictive values and their 95% confidence intervals (using the exact Clopper-Pearson method) were calculated.

4. Results

Of the 376 newborns screened over a 7-month period (June to December 2020), only 365 were valid and included in the study (figure 9). All the children were black. The mean chronological age at screening was 0.81 days (0 to 6 days) and the majority were male (201). None of the newborns had been transfused prior to screening and none were ill.

Table III. Comparison of Sickle SCAN® and capillary electrophoresis results for neonatal blood samples

Capillary electrophoresis

Sickle SCAN®		AA	SS	AS	AC	Total
	AA	218	0	5	0	223 (61,10%)
	AS	5	0	115	0	120 (32,88%)
	SS	0	21	0	0	21 (5,75%)
	AC	0	0	0	1	1 (0,27%)
Total		223 (61,10%)	21 (5,75%)	120 (32,88%)	1 (0,27%)	365 (100%)

365 newborns were screened for sickle cell disease using rapid test strips Sickle SCAN® and simultaneously for capillary electrophoresis.Overall, Sickle SCAN® identified 223 (61.10%) Hb AA, 120 (32.88%) Hb AS, 21 (5.75%) Hb SS and 1 (0.27%) Hb AC.

Table IV. Performance of the Sickle SCAN® test compared with electrophoresis capillary

Phenotype	Workforce	Results electrophoresis capillary	Results of Samples correctly tested Sickle SCAN®	Samples incorrectly tested	
Hb AA	223	A or FA	Only	218	5 (A and S)
Hb AC	1	AC	A and C	1	0
Hb AS	120	AS or FAS	A and S	115	5 (A only)
Hb SS	21	S or FS	S only	21	0
Total	365			355	10

Sickle SCAN® correctly identified the haemoglobin (Hb) phenotype in 97.26% of cases (95% CI: 95.02% - 98.68%). Sickle SCAN® correctly identified 355 out of 365 phenotypes. Only 5 samples of Hb AS were incorrectly reported by Sickle SCAN® as Hb AA and 5 samples of Hb AA were incorrectly reported as Hb AS.

Table V. Sensitivity, specificity, positive predictive value and negative predictive value and their 95% confidence intervals for the detection of HbA, HbS and HbC

		positive	negative
97,76%	96,48%	97,76%	96,48%
(94,85%-99,27%)	(91,97%-98,85%)	(94,85%-99,27%)	(91,97%-98,85%)
Hb AS 95,83%	97,96%	95,83%	97,96%
(90,54%-98,63%)	(95,30%-99,33%)	(90,54%-98,63%)	(95,30%-99,33%)
Hb SS 100,00%	100,0%	100,00%	100,0%
(83,89%-100,0%)	(98,93%-100,0%)	(83,89%-100,0%)	(98,93%-100,0%)
Hb AC 100,0%	100,00%	100,00%	100,0%
(2,50%-100,0%)	(98,99%-100,0%)	(2,50%-100,0%)	(98,99%-100,0%)

Table V shows the accuracy of detection of Hb phenotypes in neonates by Sickle SCAN® compared with gold standard capillary electrophoresis. The sensitivity, specificity, positive and negative predictive values of Sickle SCAN® were calculated. The sensitivity (97.76% [IC95%: 94.85% - 99.27%]) and specificity (96.48% [IC95%: 91.97% - 98.85%]) for the detection of Hb AA were excellent. For Hb AS, the sensitivity (95.83% [IC95%: 90.54% - 98.63%]) and specificity (97.96% [IC95%: 95.30% - 99.33%]).were also excellent. There were no false positive or false negative results for the detection of SS Hb and AC Hb, with sensitivities and specificities equal to 100%.

5. Outcome of children with sickle cell disease screened in our study

We screened 365 newborns, 21 of whom had sickle cell disease. Ten parents opted for treatment by traditional therapists for their care; 5 for the church in the hope of being cured. The parents of 6 opted for medical treatment and are being monitored to date (21 months) by the principal investigator. It should be noted that so far they have not had any vaso-occlusive seizures.

Therapeutic regimen :

☐ Compliance with vaccination schedule
☐ Antibiotic prophylaxis: Amoxicillin if febrile

☐ Multivitamins (C, E, A), folic acid, zinc
☐ Vermox every 3 months
☐ Abundant hydration
☐ A balanced diet for all ages
☐ Dress code (depending on climate)
☐ Hydrea every day depending on paraclinical data (started at 15 months due to lack of funds)

Paraclinical follow-up :

☐ Assessment of renal and hepatic function, haemogram and thick blood count every 3 months

6. Discussion

Sickle cell disease is one of the most common genetic abnormalities in the DRC. Early diagnosis remains a key factor in reducing mortality from this disease [24]. Neonatal screening makes it possible to identify children with sickle cell disease at birth or shortly afterwards, in the first few days of life and before they develop symptoms or complications. These babies can then be regularly monitored with comprehensive care and prompt management to reduce morbidity and mortality [14]. This study is the first to assess the accuracy of Sickle SCAN® in newborns in the DRC compared with capillary electrophoresis as the gold standard. The rapid test perfectly detected the Hb AC and Hb SS phenotypes diagnosed by capillary electrophoresis, and the prediction was almost perfect for Hb AS and Hb AA. Overall, the rate of discordant classification (discordant results between Sickle SCAN® and capillary electrophoresis) is estimated at 2.74% (10/365) of tests performed, higher than the 1.1% found in West Africa by Ségbana et al [16] and lower than the 4% reported in Paris (France) in the study by Nguyen-Khoa et al [21]. This rate in a diagnostic strategy could be considered acceptable, as it will be confirmed further. We therefore conclude that this rapid test is accurate and robust when used in conditions in developing countries. In a small preliminary Nigerian study of 57 adults and children, Sickle SCAN® diagnosed sickle cell disease with an error rate of 1.8% (98.2% accuracy) compared with high-performance liquid chromatography as the reference method [19].In Tanzania, Sickle SCAN® showed a sensitivity of 98.1% and a specificity of 91.1% compared with haemoglobin electrophoresis in 745 participants aged between 1 day and 20 years [20]. In the United States (Cincinnati), Sickle SCAN® had a sensitivity of 98.3% to 100% and a specificity of 92.5% to 100% for detecting the presence of Hb A, Hb S and Hb C compared with capillary electrophoresis as the reference method in 139 adults and children [18].
Sickle SCAN® has a number of potential advantages over the usual laboratory methods. Being so rapid (results available in 5 minutes), the method could contribute to routine neonatal screening for sickle cell disease in our setting, where the main barriers to implementing this neonatal screening programme, as in other low-resource areas, include the cost of diagnostic methods, lack of adequate laboratory facilities and funding. This test does not require electricity and should avoid the cost and added complexity of transporting samples and providing feedback on results [14]. It could also enable real-time communication of results and appropriate referral of newborns with sickle cell disease to specialist services. In addition, the Sickle SCAN® has a similar appearance to devices routinely used for the rapid diagnosis of other conditions such as malaria and HIV infection, with which most practitioners in resource-limited settings are familiar [14,20]. Studies carried out in various African countries reported that healthcare professionals described Sickle SCAN® as acceptable, simple, easy to interpret and giving results in less than 5 minutes [16,19]. In addition to its technical performance, Sickle SCAN® also offers socio-economic advantages as it is a low-cost test, costing US$10 compared with US$75 for haemoglobin electrophoresis.

7. Conclusion

The results of this study showed high sensitivity and specificity for newborn screening for sickle cell disease using a simple, affordable and appropriate technology. This test can be adapted at a community level to ensure early diagnosis and rapid referral for management with the aim of reducing the burden of sickle cell disease in the DRC. We conclude that Sickle SCAN® is a preferred method for neonatal screening for sickle cell disease and that its reliability is comparable to capillary electrophoresis. It is therefore ideally suited to low-resource countries.

References

1. Piel FB, Steinberg MH, Rees DC. Sickle cell disease. N Engl J Med 2017; 376 (16): 1561-73.
2. Pleasants S. Epidemiology: a moving target. Nature 2014; 515 (7526): S2-3.

3. Mukuku O, Sungu JK, Mutombo AM, Mawaw MP, Aloni NM, Wembonyama OS and Luboya NO. Albumin, copper, manganese and cobalt levels in children suffering from sickle cell anemia at Kasumbalesa, in Democratic Republic of Congo. BMC Hematol 2018; 18: 23. https://doi.org/10.1186/s12878-018-0118-z
4. Sungu JK, Mukuku O, Mutombo AM, Mawaw P, Aloni MN, Luboya ON. Trace elements in children suffering from sickle cell anemia: A case-control study. Journal of clinical laboratory analysis 2018; 32(1): e22160.
5. Ware RE, de Montalembert M, Tshilolo L, Abboud MR. Sickle cell disease. Lancet. 2017; 17:30193-9.
6. Piel FB, Patil AP, Howes RE, Nyangiri OA, Gething PW, Dewi M, Temperley WH, Williams TN, Weatherall DJ, Hay SI. Global epidemiology of sickle haemoglobin in neonates: a contemporary geostatistical model-based map and population estimates. Lancet. 2013 ;381(9861) :142-51.
7. Shongo MYP, Mukuku O. Neonatal screening for sickle cell disease in Lubumbashi, DRC. Revue de l'Infirmier Congolais. 2018 ; 2 : 62-63.

8. Modell B, Darlison M. Global epidemiology of haemoglobin disorders and derived service indicators. Bull World Health Organ. 2008;86(6):480-7.
9. Makani J, Cox SE, Soka D, Komba AN, Oruo J, Mwamtemi H, et al. Mortality in sickle cell anemia in Africa: a prospective cohort study in Tanzania. PloS one. 2011 ;6(2) : e14699.
10. Piel FB, Hay SI, Gupta S, Weatherall DJ, Williams TN. Global burden of sickle cell anemia in children under five, 2010-2050: modelling based on demographics, excess mortality, and interventions. PLoS Med. 2013;10(7): e1001484.
11. Chaturvedi S, DeBaun MR. Evolution of sickle cell disease from a life-threatening disease of children to a chronic disease of adults: the last 40 years. Am J Hematol. 2016;91(1):5- 14.
12. Platt OS, Brambilla DJ, Rosse WF, Milner PF, Castro O, Steinberg MH, et al. Mortality in sickle cell disease. Life expectancy and risk factors for early death. N Engl J Med.

1994;330(23):1639-44.

13. Quinn CT. Sickle cell disease in childhood: from newborn screening through transition to adult medical care. Pediatric clinics of North America. 2013;60(6):1363-81.

14. Williams TN. An accurate and affordable test for the rapid diagnosis of sickle cell disease could revolutionize the outlook for affected children born in resource-limited settings. BMC medicine 2015 ; 13 :238.

15. Alvarez OA, Hustace T, Voltaire M, et al. Newborn Screening for Sickle Cell Disease Using Point-of-Care Testing in Low-Income Setting. Pediatrics. 2019 ;144(4) : e20184105.

16. Segbena AY, Guindo A, Buono R, Kueviakoe I, Diallo DA, Guernec G, et al. Diagnostic accuracy in field conditions of the sickle SCAN® rapid test for sickle cell disease among children and adults in two West African settings: the DREPATEST study. BMC hematology 2018; 18: 26.

17. Kanter J, Telen MJ, Hoppe C, Roberts CL, Kim JS, Yang X. Validation of a novel point of care testing device for sickle cell disease. BMC medicine 2015 ; 13 :225.

18. McGann PT, Schaefer BA, Paniagua M, Howard TA, Ware RE. Characteristics of a rapid, point-of-care lateral flow immunoassay for the diagnosis of sickle cell disease. Am J Hematol. 2016;91(2):205-10.

19. Nwegbu MM, Isa HA, Nwankwo BB, Okeke CC, Edet-Offong UJ, Akinola NO, Adekile AD, Aneke JC, Okocha EC, Ulasi T, et al. Preliminary evaluation of a point-of-care testing device (Sickle SCAN) in screening for sickle cell disease. Hemoglobin. 2017;41(2):77-82.

20. Smart LR, Ambrose EE, Raphael KC, Hokororo A, Kamugisha E, Tyburski EA, Lam WA, Ware RE, McGann PT. Simultaneous point-of-ca]re detection of anemia and sickle cell disease in Tanzania: the RAPID study. Ann Hematol. 2018;97(2):239-46.

21. Nguyen-Khoa T, Mine L, Allaf B, Ribeil JA, Remus C, Stanislas A, Gauthereau V, Enouz S, Kim JS, Yang X, Gluckman E, Beaudeux JL, Munnich A, Girot R, Cavazzana M. Sickle SCAN™ (BioMedomics) fulfills analytical conditions for neonatal screening of sickle cell disease. Ann Biol Clin 2018; 76(4): 416-20.

22. DRC Ministry of Public Health. Health accounts report 2014. Kinshasa: PNCNS; October 2016.

23. Lwanga SK, Lemeshow S. Sample size determination in health studies: a practical manual. Geneva; World Health Organization. 1991. https://apps.who.int/iris/handle/10665/40062

24. Katamea T, Mukuku O, Luboya O, Tshilolo L, Wembonyama S. Diagnostic accuracy of the Sickle SCAN TM rapid test for neonatal screening for sickle cell disease in Lubumbashi, Democratic Republic of Congo. British Journal of Haematology 2021; 193 (Suppl. 1): 25.

Objective 2

Determine the level of acceptability of DND and the factors influencing him in the city of Lubumbashi in the DRC

Authors: *Katamea T, Mukuku O, Mutombo KA, Tshilolo LM, Luboya NO, Wembonyama SO*

Journal: *Global Journal of Medical, Pharmaceutical, and Biomedical Update*

Original article : *No GJMPBU_7_2022*

1. Summary

Introduction: Sickle cell disease is a major genetic disorder that manifests itself early in life and can lead to significant morbidity. Neonatal screening for sickle cell disease (NSCD) is one of the effective health services that has helped to reduce the burden of sickle cell disease in developed countries. Paradoxically, in sub-Saharan Africa, where the majority of newborns are born with this disease, DND programmes are almost non-existent. The aim of this study was to determine the level of acceptability of DND and the factors influencing it in the population of the city of Lubumbashi in the Democratic Republic of Congo.

Methods: Data on socio-demographic characteristics, knowledge and attitudes towards sickle cell screening were collected using a pre-tested, semi-structured questionnaire from 1 to 31 December 2020 from 2032 adults in the city of Lubumbashi.

Results: There was good awareness of sickle cell disease as a hereditary blood disorder. The DND acceptability rate was 84.50%. We found that age (p=0.002), sex (p=0.025) and religion (p=0.000) were significantly associated with DND acceptability (p<0.05).

Conclusion: This study suggests that DND is well accepted in Lubumbashi. The main obstacles to its use are probably financial and practical, rather than social or cultural.

Key words: Sickle cell disease; Neonatal screening; Acceptability; Lubumbashi.

2. Introduction

Sickle cell disease, also known as sickle cell anaemia, is a blood disorder linked to an abnormality in the structure of haemoglobin. It is caused by the production of abnormal haemoglobin, linked to a mutation in the gene coding for the synthesis of the β-globin chain, and transmitted by both father and mother (autosomal recessive disease). This characteristic leads to the production of abnormal haemoglobin S (HbS), which causes deformation of the red blood cells and disorders leading to obstruction of the blood vessels. The deformability of sickle cell red blood cells varies according to genotype and, within the same patient, according to clinical and physiological conditions [1].

The lack of reliable data in most countries makes it difficult to estimate the number of people actually affected worldwide. There are no national registries of the disease, even in developed countries that have had newborn screening programmes in place for several years (USA, UK,

France) [2]. Various estimates have been published [2-4], reporting highly variable S allele distribution frequencies depending on the region: Sub-Saharan Africa (around twenty countries with 2% to 38%), India (6 regions with 17% to 30%), Eastern Mediterranean (Saudi Arabia 1% to 29%) and Iraq (0% to 22%).In the DRC, the latest studies report a prevalence of up to 40% of the population for the heterozygous form among carriers of the sickle cell trait (otherwise known as healthy carriers), and up to 2.3% of the population for the homozygous form among sickle cell carriers. Every year, around 40,000 children with sickle cell disease are born in the DRC [5,6]. These births result in a high early mortality rate. In fact, 50-90% of these children die before the age of 5. This high mortality rate can be explained in part by the delay in diagnosing the disease, the lack of effective treatment and the limited resources of the families affected [7,8].Sickle cell disease is responsible for significant infant mortality in developing countries where there is no systematic neonatal screening programme and no comprehensive care. Neonatal screening for sickle cell anaemia (NSS) has been shown to significantly reduce sickle cell-specific infant mortality. However, the implementation of this NDS is associated with the notion of its acceptability to the target population, and this acceptability is dependent on several socio-cultural factors present from one community to another [9]. The causes attributed to illness differ between societies and within the same society. Traditional therapists certainly try to link the illness to an organic dysfunction, but most of the population's attitudes stem from the ontological meaning attributed to the illness. Is it a natural illness, an attack by a witch, an evil sent by the ancestors or a genie from the bush? The idea people have of it guides their search for remedies and their social attitudes. In Central Africa (Congo, DRC, Cameroon, Gabon), people tend to attribute illnesses, especially chronic illnesses such as sickle cell anaemia, to the aggression of a sorcerer or the malevolence of ancestral spirits. Sometimes the patient himself is considered to be an evil spirit. The search for remedies, apart from medical care of course, will then turn to the counter-sorcerer or the exorcist [10,11].

In developing countries, screening for the disease is not systematic, and is generally carried out after a first attack, which can delay the result by several months, as the main priority is to treat the severe anaemia and complications of the attack for which the child was brought to the clinic [12].

In sub-Saharan Africa, a few systematic neonatal screening pilot projects have been carried out in recent years in Ghana, Uganda, Benin and the DRC, with the support of external funding, but none, to our knowledge, has succeeded in establishing a systematic neonatal screening programme for sickle cell disease on a national scale [6,13- 16]. Unfortunately, these pilot projects have encountered a number of problems, in particular that of the acceptability of DND, both among some parents, healthcare staff and even the national authorities, for whom this screening would constitute an additional burden [17].

It is in this context that several authors consider that before any public health programme or project is implemented, a bottom-up approach is recommended, as it promotes community participation and support [18]. With this in mind, and with a view to the future introduction of a nationwide DND programme in the DRC, we proposed to carry out a survey of the acceptability of this screening among the population in our area. The aim of this study was to determine the level of acceptability of NHW and the factors influencing it in the population of the city of Lubumbashi in the DRC.

3. Materials and methods

The study was conducted in the city of Lubumbashi, in the province of Haut-Katanga. Lubumbashi is the capital of Haut-Katanga Province, in the south-east of the DRC. We conducted a descriptive cross-sectional study based on a community survey of adults. The survey was conducted between 1er and 31 December 2020. All participants gave their consent at the time of data collection. Cochran's formula for descriptive studies was used to calculate the sample size (n = z pq/d^{22}) [19], with a normal standard deviation at 95% confidence interval (1.96), an estimated prevalence of healthcare workers' knowledge of sickle cell disease of 30% [20] and a precision error at 5% (0.05). The minimum sample size calculated was 323 participants.A total of 2,450 questionnaires were distributed, 350 per commune (the city of Lubumbashi comprises 7 communes). Of the 2,450 adults invited to complete the questionnaire, 2,032 agreed to do so and were included in the study. This represented an effective participation rate of 82.9%. The data collection tool used in this study is a semi-structured questionnaire used in previous studies [21,22] which have established the validity of the questionnaire's content. This questionnaire was designed to collect information from respondents relating to socio-demographic characteristics, knowledge of DND, attitudes towards sickle cell screening policies and their attitudes towards voluntary termination of pregnancy if the participant's unborn child should be affected by sickle cell disease. The response options for closed questions were "Yes", "No" or "Don't know".Three teams of six interviewers each were formed to collect data using a multiple-choice questionnaire in French. The survey form was completed either by the interviewer if the respondent could not read or write, or by the respondent after clarification by the interviewer. A pilot study of ten selected participants was conducted to determine whether the elements questionnaire were easy to understand. The pilot interviews ensured that that no ambiguous questions were asked and to determine the time required to complete an interview. The interviews lasted an average of 25 minutes. The data obtained during the pilot interviews were not included in the final results of this study. The team was trained over three days before and after the pre-test. This covered interview techniques, the purpose of the study and ethical aspects. The principal investigator and supervisors monitored the site on a daily basis throughout the data collection period and checked that each questionnaire had been fully completed to ensure completeness and consistency. The data collected was entered into Excel 2019 and checked for inconsistencies and errors. Analyses were performed using STATA software (version 15). Frequencies and means were determined for the socio-demographic characteristics of the respondents. The distribution of each question of knowledge (e.g. causality, possibility of diagnosis in utero, after birth and at any other time) and attitude towards sickle cell screening (including before marriage, during pregnancy, after birth and reasons for each decision) were presented in figures in the form of frequencies, then cross-tabulated with the socio-demographic variables in a bivariate analysis. Pearson's Chi-square test was used to determine the association. A value of p<0.05 was considered statistically significant.

4. Results

Of a total of 2,450 respondents, 2,032 agreed to answer our questionnaire voluntarily, giving a response rate of 82.9%.

Table VI. Socio-demographic characteristics of respondents

	(N=2032)	
Age <21 years	199	9,79
21-30 years old	919	45,23
Age 31-40	694	34,15
≥41 years	220	10,83
Mean ± SD	31,0 ± 9,0	
Gender Female	1095	53,89
Male	937	46,11
Marital status Single	1103	54,28
Married	805	39,62
Separated/Divorced	124	6,10
Level of education No	72	3,54
Primary	269	13,24
Secondary	889	43,75
Higher/University	802	39,47
Professional occupation Trade	806	39,67
Employee	499	24,56
No	426	20,96
Other	301	14,81
Religion Protestant/Pentecostal	856	42,13
Catholic	816	40,16
Islamic	137	6,74
Other	223	10,97

As described in Table VI, the average age of the respondents was 31.0 ± 9.0 years and 45.23% (919/2032) of them were aged between 21 and 30 years; 53.89% were female and 46.11% male. With regard to marital status, 1103 (54.28%) of respondents said they were single, 805 (39.62%) were married and 124 (6.10%) were separated or divorced.

In terms of occupation, 806 (39.67%) said they were in trade, 499 (24.56%) were employed, 426 (20.96%) had no occupation (unemployed) and 301 (14.81%) were involved in activities other than trade. As for religion, 856 (42.13%) respondents were Pentecostal/protestants, 816 (40.16%) were Catholic, 137 (6.74%) were Islamic and 223 (10.97%) said they belonged to other religious denominations. Of the 2032 respondents, almost 40% had higher/university education, 43.75% secondary education, 13.24% primary education and 3.54% were illiterate.

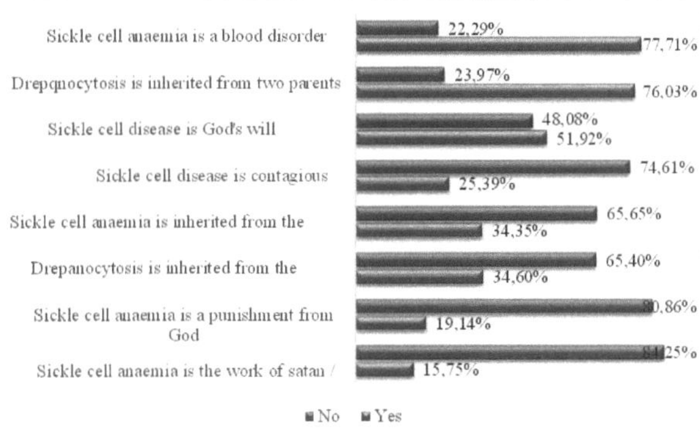

Figure 8. Respondents' general knowledge (n=2032) of sickle cell disease

Overall (Figure 8), knowledge of sickle cell anaemia as a hereditary blood disorder was good (77.71%); 1545 (76.03%) respondents knew that the disease could be inherited from both parents and 1516 (74.61%) knew that it was not contagious. As for beliefs about sickle cell anaemia, 1,055 (51.92%) said it was God's will, 389 (19.14%) said it was God's punishment, and 320 (15.75%) thought it was the work of Satan or evil spirits. Three hundred and seventy-seven people (18.55%) were aware of their status in relation to sickle cell anaemia and of these 20 (5.31%) had indicated that they were sickle cell patients (SS) and 54 (14.32%) had a sickle cell trait (AS).

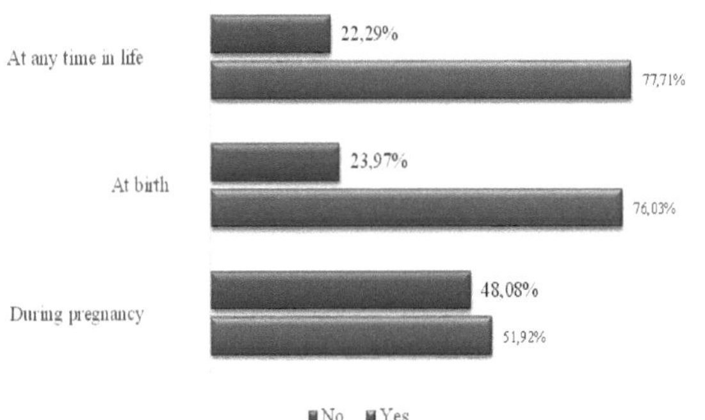

Figure 9. Respondents' (n=2032) knowledge of the sickle cell screening period

As shown in figure 9, 1584 (77.71%) respondents said that sickle cell disease can be diagnosed at any time in a person's life, 1043 (51.33%) knew that it can be diagnosed at birth (neonatal diagnosis) and 914 (44.98%) said that it can be diagnosed before birth (prenatal diagnosis).

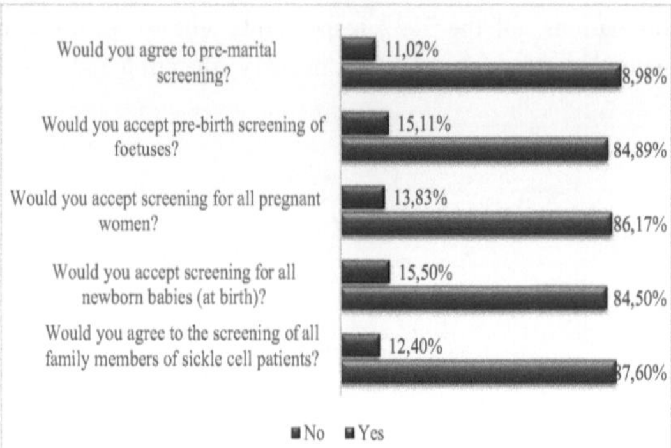

Figure 10. Attitudes of respondents (n=2032) towards sickle cell screening

In terms of respondents' attitudes to sickle cell screening, the most acceptable form of screening for sickle cell disease was pre-marital screening (88.98%), while the least acceptable was neonatal diagnosis (84.50%). Screening family members and all pregnant women was also acceptable for 87.60% and 86.17% respectively. We examined the respondents' answers concerning the termination of a pregnancy in which the foetus has sickle cell anaemia. Nearly 9 out of 10 respondents (1780/2032 or 87.60%) were against terminating the pregnancy and 12.40% (252/2032) were in favour of terminating the pregnancy. The most common reasons given for not terminating a pregnancy were religious considerations (65.71%), followed by ethical considerations (34.29%). On the other hand, for the reasons given by respondents who were in favour o f terminating the pregnancy, we noted that social considerations (marginalisation, inferiority complex) came first (49.56%), followed by economic considerations (32.46%) and cultural considerations (witchcraft) (17.98%).

Table VII. Acceptability of neonatal screening for sickle cell disease according to sociodemographic characteristics

Variable Total=2032 Yes=1717 Chi squarep-value

		n (%)		
Age <21 years	199	150 (75,38%)	14,37	0,002
21-30 years old	919	790 (85,96%)		
Age 31-40	694	589 (84,87%)		
≥41 years	220	188 (85,45%)		
Gender Male	937	773 (82,50%)	5,03	0,025
Female	1095	944 (86,21%)		
Marital status Single	1103	921 (83,50%)	2,58	0,275
Married	805	693 (86,09%)		
Divorced/Separated Level of education None/Primary	124	103 (83,06%)	2,14	0,343
	341	284 (83,28%)		
Secondary	889	763 (85,83%)		
Higher/University Religion Protestant/Pentecostal	802 856	670 (83,54%) 723 (84,46%)	95,29	0,000
Catholic	816	723 (88,60%)		
Islamic	137	77 (56,20%)		
Other Professional occupation Unemployed	223 426	194 (87,00%) 356 (83,57%)	6,88	0,075
Trade	806	665 (82,51%)		
Employee	499	437 (87,58%)		
Other activities	301	259 (86,05%)		

Table VII shows the associations between the acceptability of DND and the socio-demographic characteristics of respondents. We found that age, sex and religion were significantly associated with DND acceptability (p<0.05). However, no significant relationship was found between DND acceptability and the following variables: marital status, level of education and professional occupation. The level of acceptability of DND was 75.38%, 85.96%, 84.87% and 85.45% respectively in respondents aged <21, 21-30, 31-40 and ≥41 years. The comparison between these rates was statistically significant (X^2 =14.37; p<0.002). Respondents aged ≥21 years were more likely to accept DND than those aged <21 years.

With regard to gender, the level of acceptability of DND was statistically higher among female respondents (86.21%) than among male respondents (82.50%) (X^2 =5.03; p=0.025).

In terms of religion, the level of acceptance of the DND was 88.60%, 84.46%, 56.20% and 87.00% respectively among Catholics, Protestants/Pentecostals, Muslims and other religious denominations. The Pearson test shows a statistically significant difference between these rates (X^2 =95.29; p<0.001).

Table VIII. Factors associated with the acceptability of newborn screening for sickle cell disease

Variable	Adjusted OR	[95% Conf	Interval]	Sig	
Age <21 years old	1,00	-	-		
21-30 years old	1,95	1,32	2,87	***	
Age 31-40	1,84	1,21	2,79	***	
≥41 years	1,74	1,00	3,02	**	
Gender Male	1,00	-	-		
Female	1,31	1,00	1,72	**	
Marital status Single	1,00	-	-		
Married	1,34	0,99	1,81	*	
Divorced/Separated	1,15	0,67	1,97	*	
Level of education None/Primary	1,00	-	-		
Secondary	1,03	0,71	1,49	*	
Higher/University	0,87	0,60	1,25	*	
Religion Protestant/Pentecostal	1,00	-	-		
Catholic	1,50	1,11	2,02	***	
Islamic	0,24	0,16	0,36	***	
Other	1,25	0,80	1,95	*	
Professional activity Unemployed	1,00	-	-		
Trade	1,04	0,74	1,48	*	
Employee	1,48	0,99	2,20	*	
Other activities	1,50	0,95	2,38	*	

*** p<0.01; ** p<0.05; * p>0.05

We found that women were more likely to accept DND than men (adjusted OR=1.31 [1.00-1.72]; p=0.048). Compared with Protestants/Pentecostals, Catholics were more likely to accept DND (adjusted OR=1.50 [1.11-2.02]; p=0.009); Muslims, on the other hand, were less likely to accept DND (adjusted OR=0.24 [0.16-0.36]; p<0.001).

5. Discussion

The acceptability of NCDs is an area that has been relatively little studied. To the best of our knowledge, the present study is the first in Lubumbashi, and one of the few in the DRC and sub-Saharan Africa, to assess the population's knowledge of and attitudes towards neonatal diagnosis of sickle cell disease.The main message from this study is that the DND is readily accepted by 84.50% of the population. A prevalence rate of this magnitude is indicative of the support that a systematic DND programme would generate. This acceptance rate is relatively close to the 86.1% noted by Nnodu et al. [21] and 86% found by Oluwole et al [23] in Nigeria. Higher rates have been reported: 99% by Tubman et al [24] in Liberia and 99.7% by Odunvbun et al [25] in Nigeria. In contrast to our results, a recent study carried out in Koula-Moutou (Gabon) found an acceptability rate of 30% [20]. This study shows that there are a number of beliefs about sickle cell disease among the respondents, although the level of knowledge was good. Supernatural explanations for the cause of sickle cell disease are common in many African contexts [26]. Given that DND relies on the trust and opinion of the population, these misconceptions need to be adequately addressed not only at all levels of healthcare, but also through functional intersectoral collaboration, particularly with the media [21].

One of the main aims of the present study was to determine the factors that should be taken into account to encourage participation in DND programmes, which would maximise the cost-effectiveness of the programme once installed. Our results show that the level of acceptability of DND was associated with age and gender. In contrast to the study by Nnodu et al [21], the present study found that younger respondents (<21 years) were less supportive of DND. Female respondents were more in favour of DND than male respondents. We believe that the fact that in our African societies it is women who are mainly responsible for childcare means that they are more sensitive to child health problems than men and that they readily accept neonatal screening. Our results show that, compared with Protestants/Pentecostals, Catholics were more likely to accept DND; Muslims, on the other hand, were less likely. This finding is consistent with that of Nnodu et al [21] who found that Muslims were less supportive of DND. We believe that our results may be partly explained by the fact that a large majority of Christian churches require couples intending to be married to be screened for sickle cell anaemia before marriage. Mass mobilisation and awareness-raising efforts therefore need to be stepped up, with appeals to religious leaders to show an interest in counselling and premarital screening for sickle cell anaemia.In developed countries, DND with appropriate follow-up and care of affected children in specialised centres has led to a reduction in the mortality rate from sickle cell disease from 16% to <1% [27,28]. In developing countries, it is recognised that an unknown number of children with sickle cell disease are likely to die with the disease undiagnosed, untreated or undertreated [29]. Given that service provision in the DRC is hampered by major economic and organisational difficulties, the results of this study are an invitation to the health authorities to implement a nationwide NCD policy so that children with sickle cell disease can benefit from medical care and monitoring throughout their lives.The salient point of our study is that it is the first to address the issue of acceptability of newborn screening in the DRC. Its results provide answers to the many questions raised by the various systematic NCD projects conducted in the DRC. Its large sample (n=2032) helped to establish statistically significant associations between the acceptability of DND and the factors that appear to influence it. These associations are very useful because they help to guide policies for raising public awareness of DND and to understand the factors that influence it.A major limitation of our study is the possibility of selection bias, as our study population is exclusively urban. Thus, the results of this study could only be considered applicable to the urbanised population.Despite this limitation, the results of the current research provide an acceptable starting point for discussion on a national policy for NHW.

6. Conclusion

The present study has shown that DND is acceptable to the population in the city of Lubumbashi. This is encouraging in view of the implementation of a systematic DND programme aimed at reducing the burden of sickle cell disease in the DRC. However, the study reveals and underlines the need to raise awareness among the population in order to abandon bad beliefs about sickle cell anaemia and increase the level of acceptance among all sections of society.

References

1. Connes P. Physiopathology of sickle cell disease. In: de Montalembert, Allali S, Brousse V, Marchetti MT. Sickle cell disease in children and adolescents. Paris: Elsevier Masson; 2020.
2. Piel FB, Patil AP, Howes RE, Nyangiri OA, Gething PW, Dewi M, et al. Global epidemiology of sickle haemoglobin in neonates: a contemporary geostatistical model- based map and population estimates. Lancet 2013;381(9861):142-51.
3. Modell B, Darlison M. Global epidemiology of haemoglobin disorders and derived service indicators. Bull WHO 2008;86(6):480-7.
4. Modell B, Darlison M, Birgens H, Cario H, Faustino P, Giordano PC, et al. Epidemiology of hemoglobin disorders in Europe: an overview. Scand J Clin Lab Invest 2007;67(1):39- 69.
5. Tshilolo, L, Kafando E, Sawadogo M, coton F, Vertongen F, Ferter U and Gulbis B. (2008). Neonatal screening and clinical care programs for sickle cell disorders in sub-Saharan Africa: Lessons from pilot studies. Public Health 2008; 122(9): 933-941.
6. Tshilolo L, Aissi LM, Lukusa D, Kinsiama C, Wembonyama S, Gulbis B, Vertongen F. Neonatal screening for sickle cell anemia in the Democratic Republic of the Congo: experience from a pioneer project on 31 204 newborns. Transfus Med 2010; 20(1): 62-5;
7. Grosse, S.D., et al. Sickle cell disease in Africa: a neglected cause of early childhood mortality. American journal of preventive medicine, 2011; 41(6 Suppl 4): S398-405.
8. Kumar, A.A., et al. Evaluation of a density-based rapid diagnostic test for sickle cell disease in a clinical setting in Zambia. PloS One 2014; 9(12): e114540.

9. Katuala T.E. Multicentre survey on the acceptability of neonatal screening for sickle cell disease in Kinshasa, Democratic Republic of Congo. Faculty of Public Health, Catholic University of Louvain, 2019. Promoter: Léonard, Christian. http://hdl.handle.net/2078.1/thesis:19766.

10. Bediako SM, Neblett Jr EW. Optimism and perceived stress in sickle-cell disease: The role of an afro cultural social ethos. Journal of Black Psychology 2011 ; 37(2) : 234-253.

11. Olatunya OS, Babatola AO, Ogundare EO, Olofinbiyi BA, Lawal OA, Awoleke JO, et al. Perceptions and practice of early diagnosis of sickle cell disease by parents and physicians in a southwestern state of Nigeria. The Scientific World Journal 2020; 2020: Article ID 4801087.

12. National Institutes of Health, Consensus. Consensus conference. Newborn screening for sickle cell disease and other hemoglobinopathies. Journal of American Medical Association 1987; 258(9): 1205-1209.

13. Ohene-Frempong K, Oduro J, Tetteh H, Nkrumah F. Newborn screening for sickle cell disease in Ghana. Paediatrics. 2008, 12 : 5-7.

14. Inusa BP, Daniel Y, Lawson JO, Dada J, Matthews CE, et al. Sickle Cell Disease Screening in Northern Nigeria: The Coexistence of B- Thalassemia Inheritance. Pediat Therapeut 2015; 5: 262. Doi :10.4172/2161-0665.1000

15. Rahimy MC, Gangbo A, Ahouigan G, Alihonou E. Newborn screening for sickle cell disease in Republic of Benin. J Clin Pathol. 2009 ; 62 : 46-48.

16. Ndeezi G, Kiyaga C, Hernandez AG, Munube D, Howard TA, Ssewanyana I, et al. Burden of sickle cell trait and disease in the Uganda Sickle Surveillance Study (US3): a cross-sectional study. The Lancet Global Health 2016; 4(3): e195-e200.

17. Shongo MYP, Mukuku O. Neonatal screening for sickle cell disease in Lubumbashi, DRC. Revue de l'Infirmier Congolais. 2018 ; 2 : 62-63.

18. Carlton J, Griffiths HJ, Horwood AM, Mazzone PP, Walker R, Simonsz HJ. Acceptability of childhood screening: a systematic narrative review. Public health 2021; 193: 126-138.

19. DRC Ministry of Public Health. Rapport des comptes de la santé 2014. Kinshasa: PNCNS; October 2016.

20. Mombo LE, Makosso LK, Bisseye C, Mbacky K, Setchell JM, Edou A. Acceptability of neonatal sickle cell disease screening among parturient women at the Paul Moukambi Regional Hospital in rural Eastern Gabon, Central Africa. African Journal of Reproductive Health 2021; 25(3): 72-77.

21. Nnodu OE, Adegoke SA, Ezenwosu OU, Emodi II, Ugwu NI, Ohiaeri CN, et al. A Multi-centre Survey of Acceptability of Newborn Screening for Sickle Cell Disease in Nigeria. Cureus 2018; 10(3): e2354.

22. Wonkam A, Njamnshi AK, Mbanya D, Ngogang J, Zameyo C, Angwafo FF. Acceptability of prenatal diagnosis by a sample of parents of sickle cell anemia patients in Cameroon (sub-Saharan Africa). Journal of genetic counseling 2011; 20(5): 476-485.

23. Oluwole EO, Adeyemo TA, Osanyin GE, Odukoya OO, Kanki PJ, Afolabi BB (2020) Feasibility and acceptability of early infant screening for sickle cell disease in Lagos, Nigeria-A pilot study. PLoS ONE 15(12): e0242861.

24. Tubman VN, Marshall R, Jallah W, Guo D, Ma C, Ohene-Frempong K, et al. Newborn Screening for Sickle Cell Disease in Liberia: A pilot study. Pediatr Blood Cancer. 2016; 63 (4): 671-676.

25. Odunvbun ME, Okolo AA, Rahimy CM. Newborn screening for sickle cell disease in a Nigerian hospital. Public health 2008; 122(10): 1111-1116.

26. Marsh VM, Kamuya DM and Molyneux SS. 'All her children are born that way': gendered experiences of stigma in families affected by sickle cell disorder in rural Kenya. Ethn Health 2011; 16(4-5): 343-59. https://doi.org/10.1080/13557858.2010.541903.

27. Komba, A. N., Makani, J., Sadarangani, M., et al. (2009). Malaria as a cause of morbidity and mortality in children with homozygous sickle cell disease on the coast o f Kenya. Clinical Infectious Diseases, 49(2), 216- 22.

28. Streetly A, Latinovic R, Hall K, Henthorn J. (2009). Implementation of universal newborn bloodspot screening for sickle cell disease and other clinically significant haemoglobinopathies in England: screening results for 2005-7. Journal of Clinical Pathology, 62(1), 26- 30.

29. Makani J, Cox SE, Soka D, Komba AN, Oruo J, Mwamtemi H, et al (2011) Mortality in Sickle Cell Anemia in Africa: A Prospective Cohort Study in Tanzania. PLoS ONE 6(2) : e14699. https://doi.org/10.1371/journal.pone.0014699

Objective 3: Determine the prevalence of sickle cell disease in Lubumbashi, Democratic Republic of Congo
Authors: *Tina Katamea, Olivier Mukuku, Stanis O. Wembonyama*

Journal: *British Journal of Haematology*

Original article: *2021; 193 (Suppl. 1): 31*

1. Summary

Introduction: Sickle cell disease is an autosomal recessive haemoglobinopathy. It affects around 2% of newborns in certain sub-Saharan African countries. In most patients, the incidence of complications can be reduced if screening takes place at birth. This study was carried out to determine the prevalence of sickle cell disease in a population of newborns in Lubumbashi, in the Democratic Republic of Congo.

Methods: This prospective cross-sectional study was conducted from June to December 2020 among newborns in 9 health facilities in the city of Lubumbashi, Democratic Republic of Congo. Blood samples from newborns were examined by capillary electrophoresis.

Results: Of a total of 538 newborns screened for sickle cell disease, 369 (68.59%; CI95%: 64.48% - 72.49%) were AA; 141 (26.21%; CI95%: 22.54% - 72.49%) were AA.
30.14%) were AS; 27 (5.01%; IC95%: 3.33% - 7.22%) were AS.

SS and 1 (0.19%; CI95%: 0.00% - 1.03%) neonates were AC.
Conclusion: This study determined the prevalence of sickle cell disease during neonatal screening in Lubumbashi. Premarital counselling is essential to reduce the prevalence of this haemoglobinopathy, which is very high (5.01% of Hb SS). Systematic newborn screening in all maternity units in the country would help to assess the prevalence at national level and improve the quality of life of children with sickle cell disease.

Key words: Sickle cell disease; Neonatal screening; Prevalence; Newborn; Lubumbashi.

2. Introduction

Sickle cell disease is an inherited haemoglobinopathy resulting from the substitution of valine for the glutamic amino acid in the sixth position of the beta-globin chain [1]. Sickle cell trait is inherited in an autosomal recessive pattern. Phenotypically, only individuals with double recessive sickle cell disease genes (homozygous SS) manifest the disease, while heterozygotes (AS) are called healthy carriers.
According to D. Diallo, Africa is the continent most affected, with 200,000 newborns with sickle cell anaemia each year [2]. This represents around 66.6% of children born with haemoglobinopathies worldwide. The lack of reliable data in most countries makes it difficult to estimate the number of people actually affected worldwide. There are no national registries of the disease, even in developed countries that have had newborn screening programmes in place for several years (United States, United Kingdom, France) [3]. Various estimates have

been published [3-5], reporting highly variable S allele distribution frequencies depending on the region: Sub-Saharan Africa (around twenty countries with frequencies ranging from 2% to 38%), India (6 regions with frequencies ranging from 17% to 30%), the Eastern Mediterranean (Arabia, Saudi Arabia, South Africa, etc.) and the Middle East.
Saudi Arabia [1% to 29%] and Iraq [0% to 22%]).
In the DRC, the latest studies report a prevalence of up to 40% of the population for the heterozygous form among carriers of the sickle cell trait (otherwise known as healthy carriers), and up to 2.3% of the population for the homozygous form among sickle cell carriers. Every year, around 40,000 children with sickle cell disease are born in the DRC [6]. According to reports from Ghana, an estimated 15,000 children are born with sickle cell disease every year [7]. In Benin, the prevalence of sickle cell trait is estimated at 25% [8], while in Nigeria it varies from 24 to 25% [9,10].In all these African countries, the concentration of the sickle cell trait has been found to be highest in specified subpopulations [2,9,10], probably due to conservative tribal marriages. The autosomal recessive inheritance pattern assumed by the sickle cell trait, however, predicts changes in population-level dynamics, ease of movement and intertribal marriages that would alter the distribution of the sickle cell trait within these communities [11]. Available data on the prevalence of sickle cell disease in a population of newborns in Lubumbashi are based on a preliminary survey conducted by Shongo and Mukuku in 2017 [12]. According to this study, the prevalence of sickle cell disease among newborns was 15.61% (3.47% of newborns were carriers of a major sickle cell syndrome and 12.14% were heterozygous sickle cell AS) [12]. In the light of advances in health interventions, screening and premarital counselling of the population, it is assumed that the distribution of the sickle cell trait among African populations may be strategically modified. We hypothesised that a current survey of the prevalence of sickle cell disease in Lubumbashi would be informative given that 3 years have already passed since the last study, which was only preliminary [12]. This study was therefore conducted to provide an update on the prevalence of sickle cell disease in the city of Lubumbashi, DRC.

3. Materials and methods

3.1. Scope and type of study

This was a prospective, descriptive, cross-sectional study involving newborns. We conducted neonatal screening for sickle cell disease in the maternity wards of 9 health facilities in the city of Lubumbashi, Democratic Republic of Congo, from June to December 2020. These were Cliniques Universitaires, Jason Sendwe Provincial Reference General Hospital, Katuba Reference General Hospital, Kamalondo Reference General Hospital, Kenya Reference General Hospital, Kisanga Health Zone Hospital, Ruashi Military Hospital, Camp Vangu Military Hospital and Saint François Hospital.

3.2. Population studied

This study focused on newborns in the maternity units mentioned above and the screening involved newborns aged 6 days or less. Informed consent was sought from any woman who agreed to have her newborn screened. The study excluded any newborn with any disease diagnosed during the maternity stay, any transfused newborn and any newborn whose mothers did not agree to participate in the study. Demographic data and contact details were collected prior to blood sampling using a pre-established form and were then entered into a database in Microsoft Excel format.

3.3. Sampling

The Cochran formula for descriptive studies was used to calculate the sample size (n = z pq/d^{22}) [13], with a 95% confidence interval standard deviation (1.96), an estimated sickle cell prevalence of 3.47% [12] and a precision error of 2.5% (0.025). The minimum sample size calculated was 206 participants. Taking into account a 20% non-response rate, a sample size of 248 was calculated, but 538 newborns were finally recruited for the study.

3.4. Conduct of the survey

Health education was provided prior to obtaining consent for a newborn to be screened. The duration of the education was approximately 30 minutes and depended on the mothers' questions. Health education on sickle cell disease was provided through a short interview with a group of mothers. The information included the origin of sickle cell disease, the different types of sickle cell status, the importance of clinic visits and healthy lifestyles. The training was given in Swahili and/or French to ensure understanding. The results of the sickle cell screening were communicated to all the mothers. Children who tested positive for sickle cell disease were referred to the paediatrician (principal investigator) for further follow-up and advice.

3.5. Sample collection and analysis techniques

A maximum of 500 µl of blood sample was taken in microtainer tubes of ethylene diamine tetra acetic acid (EDTA) from the venipuncture of the back of the hand of each newborn in the selected health facilities. The newborns' blood samples were then stored in a cool box at 5° C and flown to the laboratory at Monkole Hospital in Kinshasa (DRC), where capillary electrophoresis was performed using a new-generation machine, the Capillarys 2 Flex Piercing System [Sebia SA, France].The Sebia capillary electrophoresis method involves several steps. Firstly, the primary tubes containing the previously prepared red blood cells are placed on the injection point of the rack. The barcodes are placed facing the reading window. After injection of the At the sample rack, the automated system reads the barcodes on the primary sample tubes. The samples are then haemolyzed and diluted with the haemolysing solution in the reagent cups, rinsing the sampling needle between each dilution. The capillaries are washed before the haemolysed samples are injected into the capillaries, and the injection is carried out at the anode by suction. The different haemoglobin fractions then migrate through the capillaries in a basic medium (pH 9.4), allowing them to be separated and detected directly at the cathode. The migration, which lasts around 14 minutes, takes place at a high constant voltage (several thousand volts) and at a temperature controlled by the Peltier effect. The various haemoglobin peaks are read at 415 nm, corresponding to the wavelength of maximum absorption of haemoglobin. All these steps result in electrophoretic tracings or profiles which are then interpreted by the biologist.

3.6. Statistical analysis

Statistical analyses were performed using STATA 16 software (Stata Corp, College Station, TX). Proportions were calculated for the different haemoglobin types and results were presented with a two-sided 95% confidence interval using the Wilson score method with continuity correction.

4. Results

Neonatal screening for sickle cell disease was carried out for 7 months (June to December 2020). As this was a study phase and neonatal screening for sickle cell disease is not a health policy in the DRC, blood samples were collected according to the availability of resources and for a few hours each day. 600 participants were selected and 62 mothers had refused to give consent for their newborns to be screened.A total of 538 blood samples were taken and analysed, of which 286 (53.16%) were boys and 252 (46.84%) girls. All the children were black. The mean chronological age at screening was 0.62 days (0 to 6 days). None of the newborns had been transfused prior to screening.

Table IX: Haemoglobin phenotypes of 538 newborns

Haemoglobin phenotypes Workforce Percentage (IC95%)

	(n=538)	
AA	369	68,59 (64,48 - 72,49)
AS	141	26,21 (22,54 - 30,14)
SS	27	5,01 (3,33 - 7,22)
AC	1	0,19 (0,00 - 1,03)

The phenotypes were as follows: 369 (68.59%; CI95%: 64.48% - 72.49%) newborns were AA; 141 (26.21%; CI95%: 22.54% - 30.14%) newborns were AS; 27 (5.01% ; IC95%: 3.33% - 7.22%) newborns were SS and 1 (0.19%; IC95%: 0.00% - 1.03%) newborns were AC.

5. Discussion

These results, although limited to the city, provide some information on the prevalence of sickle cell disease in newborns in Lubumbashi. We carried out screening in 9 reference maternity units in Lubumbashi. During the study period, 600 mothers were made aware of the need to screen their newborns for sickle cell disease, and 538 (89.7%) of them accepted. We consider that this acceptance rate is fairly significant and would justify the implementation of systematic neonatal screening for sickle cell disease throughout the country. This study shows that 5.01% of newborns were SS (homozygous sickle cell disease), 26.21% were AS (sickle cell trait carriers) and 0.19% were AC (C trait carriers). These results are striking, given the high prevalence of sickle cell disease (5.01% SS Hb) found in the neonatal population in

Lubumbashi. This study comes just after the preliminary study recently published by Shongo and Mukuku [8] in which a neonatal screening for sickle cell disease carried out on 173 newborns screened in the maternity wards of 3 health facilities in the city of Lubumbashi reported 12.14% Hb AS and 3.47% Hb SS. As in the present study, these authors did not find any cases of composite SC heterozygosity in their series, probably because of the low prevalence of Hb C in the Congolese population in general [6].

In the DRC, two other similar studies had already been carried out [6,14]. The first, involving 520 newborns in 5 health facilities in the city of Kisangani, found that 23.3% of newborns were carriers of the sickle cell trait and 0.96% of homozygous sickle cell SS [14]. The second, carried out in a series of 31204 newborns recruited throughout France, reported that 16.9% of newborns were carriers of the sickle cell trait and 1.4% of homozygous SS sickle cells [6]. The latter noted that there was no statistically significant difference between the country's different ethnolinguistic groups, but that a high prevalence of the beta S gene was noted in tribes where the prevalence of malaria is high [6]. A previous study, carried out in the Great Lakes region (Burundi, Rwanda and the eastern part of the DRC) in 4 maternity units in a series of 1825 newborns, found 0.11% of major sickle cell syndrome and 3.28% of sickle cell trait (SCD). The presence of Hb C was noted in 4 newborns (i.e. 0.22%) [15]. In Gabon, 143 children were heterozygous (15.10%) and 17 homozygous (1.80%) in a series of 947 newborns recruited in two maternity hospitals in Libreville [16]. In Nigeria, in the city of Benin, Odunvbun et al [17], in a series of 628 newborns recruited, found that 133 (20.6%) were AS, 7 (1.1%) were homozygous, and the rest were heterozygous. were AC, 18 (2.8%) were SS and 1 (0.2%) was SC. In view of these results, it is preferable to introduce systematic screening of all newborns rather than targeted screening (limited to screening newborns of mothers who know their haemoglobin phenotypes). Odunvbun et al [17] pointed out that mothers' lack of knowledge of their own phenotype may have led to the high level of marriage among sickle cell trait carriers, resulting in the high prevalence of sickle cell disease in their community. The impact of information and awareness-raising about sickle cell anaemia on the general population, and particularly on young adolescents and adults, is very significant. This is illustrated by the example of a long information and education campaign carried out in Bahrain in the Middle East, which reduced the rate of carriers of major sickle cell syndrome by 60% in 18 years [18].Sickle cell anaemia remains unknown and ignored by the Congolese population in general, and is most often equated with witchcraft. This turns patients away from hospitals, often sending them to charlatans. Many people are unaware of the disease, which leads to patients being stigmatised, rejected and mocked by their peers and those around them. Patients and their families are left to fend for themselves, living in conditions of great suffering. unbearable and unacceptable physical and psychological suffering. The financial burden of sickle cell anaemia leaves families breathless and often broken. The various methods of screening for sickle cell anaemia are almost non-existent in hospitals in Lubumbashi; only a few health centres or private laboratories offer them.

6. Conclusion

Sickle cell disease is widespread among newborns in Lubumbashi. This study determined the prevalence of sickle cell disease during newborn screening in Lubumbashi. Premarital counselling is essential to reduce the prevalence of this haemoglobinopathy, which is very high (5.01% of Hb SS). Systematic newborn screening in all maternity units in the country would help to assess prevalence at national level and improve the quality of life of children with sickle cell disease.

References

1. Mukuku O, Sungu JK, Mutombo AM, Mawaw PM, Aloni MN, Wembonyama SO, Luboya ON. Albumin, copper, manganese and cobalt levels in children suffering from sickle cell anemia at Kasumbalesa, in Democratic Republic of Congo. BMC hematology 2018; 18(1): 1-5.

2. Diallo D, Tchernia G. Sickle Cell Disease in Africa. Curre Opin Hematol. 2002, 9 (2): 111-116.

3. Piel FB, Patil AP, Howes RE, Nyangiri OA, Gething PW, Dewi M, et al. Global epidemiology of sickle haemoglobin in neonates: a contemporary geostatistical model- based map and population estimates. Lancet 2013;381(9861):142-51.

4. Modell B, Darlison M. Global epidemiology of haemoglobin disorders and derived service indicators. Bull WHO 2008;86(6):480-7.

5. Modell B, Darlison M, Birgens H, Cario H, Faustino P, Giordano PC, et al. Epidemiology of haemoglobin disorders in Europe: an overview. Scand J Clin Lab Invest 2007;67(1):39- 69.

6. Tshilolo L, Aissi LM, Lukusa D, Kinsiama C, Wembonyama S, Gulbis B, Vertongen F. Neonatal screening for sickle cell anaemia in the Democratic Republic of the Congo: experience from a pioneer project on 31 204 newborns. Transfus Med 2010; 20(1): 62-5.

7. Ohene-Frempong Kwaku & Oduro, Joseph & Tetteh, Hannah & Nkrumah, Fk. Screening Newborns for Sickle Cell Disease in Ghana. Pediatrics. 121. 10.1542/peds.2007- 2022UUU.

8. Rahimy MC, Gangbo A, Ahouignan G, Adjou R, Deguenon C, Goussanou S, Alihonou E: Effect of a comprehensive clinical care programme on disease course in severely ill children with sickle cell anemia in a sub-Saharan Africa setting. Blood. 2003, 102 : 834-838.

9. Serjeant GR: Mortality of sickle cell disease in Africa. British Medical Journal. 2005, 330: 342-433.

10. Akinjanju OO: Sickle cell disorders. The Nigeria Family Practice. 1994, 3: 24-30.

11. Cvalli-Sforza LL, Menozzi P, Piazza A. The history and geography of human genes. Princeton, New Jersey, USA. 1994, Princeton University Press, 1088.

12. Shongo MYP, Mukuku O. (2018). Neonatal screening for sickle cell disease in Lubumbashi, RDC. Revue de l'Infirmier Congolais. 2018 ; 2 : 62-63.

13. Lwanga SK, Lemeshow S. Sample size determination in health studies: a practical manual. Geneva; WHO. 1991. https://apps.who.int/iris/handle/10665/40062 Accessed 20 May 2020.

14. Agasa B, Bosunga K, Opara A, Tshilumba K, Dupont E, Vertongen F, Cotton F, Gulbis B. Prevalence of sickle cell disease in a northeastern region of the Democratic Republic of

Congo: what impact on transfusion policy? J Med Screen. 2007; 14(3): 113-6.
15. Mutesa L, Boemer F, Ngendahayo L, Rulisa S, Rusingiza EK, Cwinya-Ay N, Mazina D, Kariyo PC, Bours V, Schoos R. Neonatal screening for sickle cell disease in Central Africa: a study of 1825 newborns with a new enzyme-linked immunosorbent assay test. Public Health. 2008; 122(9): 933-41.

16. Vierin Nzame Y, Boussougou Bu Badinga I, Koko J, Blot Ph, Moussavou A. Screening neonatal sickle cell disease in Gabon. Médecine d'Afrique Noire 2012; 59 (2): 95-99.

17. Odunvbun ME, Okolo AA, Rahimy CM. Newborn screening for sickle cell disease in a Nigerian hospital. Public Health 2008; 122 (10): 1111-1116.
18. Al Arrayed S. Campaign to control genetic blood diseases in Barhain. Community Genet 2005; 8(1): 52-55.

Objective 4: To assess health professionals' knowledge of sickle cell disease and neonatal screening in Lubumbashi, Democratic Republic of Congo.

Authors: *Tina Katamea, Olivier Mukuku, Patient Dinanga Nzala, Bénédicte Malonda Nsasi, Emery Kanyinda Ibeki, Alex B. Katende, André K. Mutombo, Charles Wembonyama Mpoy, Oscar Numbi Luboya, Stanis Okitotsho Wembonyama*

Journal: *Journal Hematology and Clinical Research*

Original article : *2021 ;5 : 015-020. 2021;1(2):1-7.*

1. Summary

Introduction: Sickle cell disease is an autosomal recessive haemoglobinopathy. Despite its high prevalence, there are still gaps in healthcare professionals' knowledge of this disease. The aim of this study was to assess healthcare professionals' knowledge of sickle cell disease and its neonatal screening.

Methods: This was a descriptive, cross-sectional study involving 465 healthcare providers (doctors and nurses) who responded to two closed, self-administered questionnaires in December 2020. Performance was tested in terms of mean score and proportions of correct answers for each questionnaire topic.

Results: Overall, the study reported 7.96% good knowledge of sickle cell disease and 23.66% good or excellent knowledge of neonatal screening for sickle cell disease. There was a statistical association between better performance and medical title: doctors had better knowledge than nurses.

Conclusion: This study shows gaps in knowledge among healthcare providers. These results suggest that there is scope for training in sickle-cell anaemia as a whole, in order to ensure a competent healthcare workforce in an environment highly affected by this disease.

Key word : Sickle cell disease; Knowledge; Health professionals; Neonatal screening; Lubumbashi.

2. Introduction

Sickle cell disease is an inherited red blood cell disorder characterised by the presence of abnormal haemoglobin S, either in homozygous form (Hb SS) or in association with other abnormal haemoglobins such as Hb SC and Hb Sβ-Thal [1]. The disease is characterised by chronic haemolysis, chronic inflammation, immune deficiency, a heterogeneous clinical phenotype and visceral involvement. The pathogenic mechanism in sickle cell disease is mainly due to chronic inflammation associated with oxidative stress [2]. In this condition, red blood cells have a tendency to deform into a crescent shape (sickle shape) under certain conditions, and clinical manifestations include chronic anaemia, painful vaso-occlusive crises, acute chest syndrome, bone and osteoarticular damage, stroke, priapism, hepato-biliary, cardiac and renal damage, and even early mortality [1,3,4].

The DRC is one of the three countries most affected by sickle cell disease in the world (after Nigeria and India) [5]; in some regions, sickle cell disease affects more than 2% of newborns [6-9].The World Health Organisation (WHO) estimates that 70% of sickle cell disease deaths in Africa are preventable through simple, cost-effective interventions such as early identification of affected individuals through neonatal screening and subsequent provision of comprehensive care [10,11]. Neonatal screening for sickle cell disease (NSCD) was recommended by a consensus conference on haemoglobinopathies in the USA in 1987 [12]. In the DRC, NCD has not yet been implemented as part of systematic or sustainable national strategies [13,14].

The aim of DND is twofold: (i) to identify and educate families with sickle cell disease, sickle cell trait and other haemoglobin variants; and (ii) to provide appropriate interventions to reduce mortality [15].Knowledge of sickle cell disease is one way of preventing and controlling this scourge, as healthcare professionals will be better equipped to make informed decisions about interventions to control the disease [16]. Although the WHO recommends educating the population as a means of reducing mortality from sickle cell disease [17], and despite the large number of people with sickle cell disease, the level of knowledge about sickle cell disease is still low. In the DRC, various studies have reported poor knowledge of sickle cell disease among students and the general population [18-20].

As the recipient of screening results, the healthcare provider is the key player in the diagnosis of sickle cell disease. It is the healthcare provider who is the first to receive a request for information and who must decide whether or not to undertake appropriate screening, in agreement with the patient. Healthcare professionals can make an effective contribution to raising awareness, informing and motivating the public about newborn screening for sickle cell disease. [15,21,22]

Increasing the education of healthcare providers to acquire basic knowledge is a major challenge in relation to this condition, in order to actively help those affected to avoid complications and improve their quality of life [16].

Health professionals' knowledge of sickle cell disease [18-20] and its neonatal screening [15,21,22] has been studied elsewhere, but this particular area has not yet been the subject of research in our setting. The aim of this study was to assess healthcare professionals' basic knowledge of sickle cell disease and its DNN in the city of Lubumbashi, with a view to developing updating and further training programmes.

3. Materials and methods

3.1. Scope and type of study

This descriptive cross-sectional survey was conducted in Lubumbashi, a city in the south of Haut-Katanga Province in the Democratic Republic of Congo. Lubumbashi is the capital of the province, with an estimated population of 2,478,262 million. The city is a focal point in terms of health services for the whole Province and surrounding Provinces. Doctors and nurses from various health facilities in the town formed the study population. The exclusion criteria consisted of the absence of a health care professional in the study population. health, on the day of data collection, refusal to participate in the study and submission of at least one incompletely completed questionnaire. The study took place in health centres (CS), hospitals, private clinics (CP) and the Cliniques Universitaires de Lubumbashi (CUL). We used multi-stage sampling. At the first stage, concerning the public facilities, we carried out an exhaustive sampling of all the hospitals and university clinics in Lubumbashi; we then carried out a random selection of the various public (25) and private (30) health facilities (CSs and CPs). At the second stage, by reasoned choice, we selected 5 health facilities per category (CS, hospitals, CP) with a minimum of 50 deliveries per month, i.e. 16 health facilities. The data were collected from 1 to 31 December 2020.

The interviewers recruited received training, covering the context of the current survey, detailed interpretation of the survey instruments and a mock survey test. Finally, a total of 10 interviewers were recruited. The interviewers explained the purpose and procedure of the study and obtained informed consent from each respondent before asking them to complete the questionnaires. On average, the survey lasted between 10 and 15 minutes.

A pilot study was conducted with 16 health professionals from 2 health facilities (CUL and HPGR Jason Sendwe). Participants were asked to complete the questionnaires and provide feedback on the relevance, clarity and difficulty of the questionnaire items. The participants expressed no difficulties with the questionnaires and this led to their adoption for the survey itself.

3.2. Data collection instruments and quality control

In order to collect data on knowledge of sickle cell disease, we adapted and used the "DFConhecimento" instrument developed and validated by Diniz et al [16], which contains a series of 13 main questions relating to the pathophysiology, clinical aspects and therapeutic aspects of sickle cell disease patients.

The questionnaire was closed and self-administered, with 4 to 6 assertions for each question, of which only one was considered correct. Respondents were given the option of selecting "Don't know" to discourage guesswork. To calculate the respondent's total score, 1 point was awarded for each item answered correctly and 0 points for an incorrect answer. The scores ranged from 0 to 13. To calculate the final score for the instrument, we used the sum of the correct responses, taking into account the following ranges of knowledge points: 12-13 corresponding to an accuracy of more than 90% (excellent knowledge); 8-11 corresponding to an accuracy of 60% to 89% (good knowledge); and ≤ 7 corresponding to less than 59% accuracy (poor knowledge) [16].

Regarding neonatal screening, a 4-item questionnaire developed by Walter et al [21] was adapted in our study to measure healthcare providers' knowledge of neonatal screening for sickle cell disease. The questionnaire was closed and self-administered with 2 assertions for each question, of which only one was considered correct. The knowledge questions included the following items: 1) How is sickle cell disease inherited? (Correct answer: autosomal recessive); 2) Is the sickle cell trait detected by neonatal screening? (Correct answer: yes); 3) True or false?4) True or false: sickle cell anaemia can be diagnosed by ordering a complete blood count or a red blood cell index (Correct answer: false). Each knowledge question (four in total) was given a value of '1' for a correct answer and '0' for an incorrect answer. Participants with scores of 0 to 2 were grouped into a total score category of 'poor' knowledge. Those with a score of 3 were grouped into a 'good' knowledge category. Those with scores of 4 were grouped into a 'perfect' knowledge category.

3.3. Sampling and data collection

This study consisted of interviewing health professionals (doctors and nurses) working in paediatrics in various CS (Light, Yahweh Rafa, CPP, Shaloom, Saint Clément), HGR (Kampemba, Katuba, Kenya, Kisanga, Sendwe), CUL and CP (Saint François, Holiness, Baume de Galade, Hope, Mane cachée) in the city of Lubumbashi, selected by random draw. In each health facility surveyed, the healthcare professionals present during the survey period were approached and invited to take part in the survey (204 doctors and 261 nurses). Cochran's formula for descriptive studies was used to calculate the sample size (n = z pq/d)[22][23] , with a normal standard deviation at 95% confidence interval (1.96), an estimated prevalence of healthcare workers' knowledge of sickle cell disease of 34% [21] and a precision error at 5% (0.05). The minimum sample size calculated was 345 participants. Taking into account a 20% non-response rate, a sample size of 414 was calculated. In total, 500 questionnaires were distributed and 487 were returned on site. Of the questionnaires returned, 465 contained no missing items and were included for further analysis (Figure 11). This represented an effective participation rate of 93%.

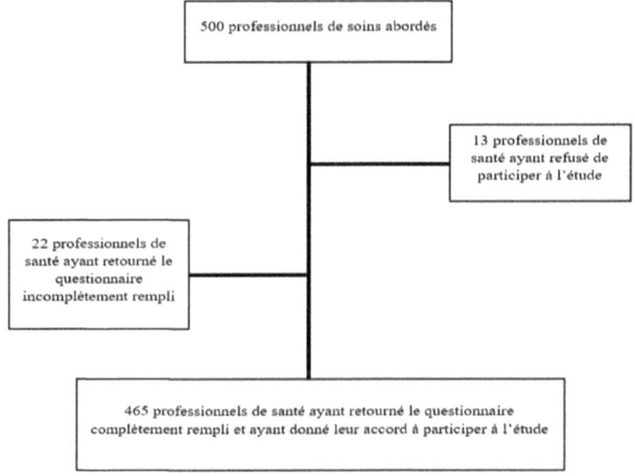

Figure 11. Recruitment of participants

3.4. Data analysis

The following variables were used to characterise the participants: age, sex, type of health facility where they worked, years of clinical practice and additional training related to sickle cell disease. The data collected was entered into Excel 2019 and checked for inconsistencies and errors. Analyses were carried out using STATA software (version 15). Data analysis included descriptive statistical calculations, frequencies and Pearson Chi-square and Fisher exact calculations to determine significance. Proportions were calculated for categorical variables and results were presented as percentages with a 95% confidence interval using Wilson score limits. Demographic and professional variables (age, sex, medical qualification, type of health training, professional experience, whether or not they had attended a session of further education on sickle cell disease in the last two years) were analysed to determine whether participants had significantly different knowledge scores. A value of p<0.05 was considered statistically significant.

4. Results

Table X. Demographic and professional characteristics of respondents

Variable Workforce Percentage

	(n=465)	
Age (years) 20-29	151	32,47
30-39	208	44,73
≥40	106	22,80
Mean ± SD	34,16 ± 8,18	
Gender Female	233	50,11
Male	232	49,89
Medical title Doctor	204	43,87
Nurse	261	56,13
Type of health facility CS	81	17,42
HGR	163	35,05
Private clinic	156	33,55
University Clinics	65	13,98
Clinical experience (years) ≤5	245	52,69
6-10	122	26,24
>10	98	21,07
Mean ± SD	7,57 ± 7,26	
Sickle cell disease training over the last 2 years No	349	75,05
Yes	116	24,95

HGR: Hôpital Général de Référence; **CS:** Centre de Santé; **SD:** standard deviation ;

N: number; **%:** percentage.

A total of 465 healthcare providers completed the survey, of whom 204 (43.87%) were doctors and 261 (56.13%) nurses. The average age of the respondents was 34.16 ± 8.18 years, and 50.11% were female (a sex ratio of 1). A third (33.55%) of respondents were working in private clinics. Respondents had an average number of years of clinical experience of 7.57 ± 7.26 years, and only around 25% had reported attending a training session on sickle cell disease in the two years preceding the survey.

Table XI. Percentages of respondents with correct answers to questions on the various themes related to sickle cell disease

Topics of questions asked	Workforce (n=465)	% (IC95%)
Definition of newborn screening	273	58,7 (54,2 - 63,1)
Definition of sickle cell disease	363	78,1 (74,1 - 81,6)
Sickle cell phenotyping	411	88,4 (85,2 - 91,0)
Sickle cell trait	74	15,9 (12,9 - 19,5)
Clinical manifestations of sickle cell disease	54	11,6 (9,0 - 14,8)
Vaso-occlusive seizures	214	46,0 (41,5 - 50,6)
Factors promoting sickle cell disease in red blood cells	160	34,4 (30,2 - 38,8)
Warning signs	72	15,5 (12,5 - 19,1)
Medicines used in the prevention and/or treatment of sickle cell disease	86	18,5 (15,2 - 22,3)
Use of antibiotics	57	12,3 (9,6 - 15,6)
Health of adolescents with sickle cell disease	143	30,8 (26,7 - 35,1)
Pregnancy and contraception	97	20,9 (17,4 - 24,8)
Care to prevent leg ulcers	143	30,8 (26,7 - 35,1)

The average score obtained by respondents was 4.6±1.9 out of a total of 13 points. The proportions of professionals giving correct answers reached over 58% for three themes (neonatal screening, definition and phenotyping of sickle cell disease). For the other themes, the correct response rates ranged from 11.6% to 46.0%.

Table XII. Percentages of respondents with correct answers to knowledge questions

Question (bonne réponse)	Type de FOSA		Total (N=465)	p-value
	Publique (n=309)	Privée (n=156)		
Quel est le mode d'hérédité (mode de transmission) de la drépanocytose ? (Autosomique récessive)	75 (24,27%)	21 (13,46%)	96 (20,65%)	0,009
Le trait drépanocytaire est-il détecté par le dépistage néonatal ? (Oui)	188 (60,84%)	96 (61,54%)	284 (61,08%)	0,964
La drépanocytose survient uniquement chez les personnes d'origine afro-américaine. (Faux)	229 (74,11%)	101 (64,74%)	330 (70,97%)	0,035
La drépanocytose peut être diagnostiquée en demandant une formule sanguine complète ou un comptage des globules rouges. (Faux)	105 (33,98%)	61 (39,10%)	166 (35,70%)	0,324

The percentages of correct answers to the knowledge questions were calculated. We noted statistically higher proportions of public health facility providers than private health facility providers regarding the mode of inheritance of sickle cell disease (24.27% versus 13.46%; p=0.009) and whether sickle cell disease occurs only in people of African-American origin (74.11% versus 64.74%; p=0.035). As for the question of whether neonatal screening detects the sickle cell trait, we noted that 61% of respondents answered correctly, whatever the type of health facility (p=0.964).

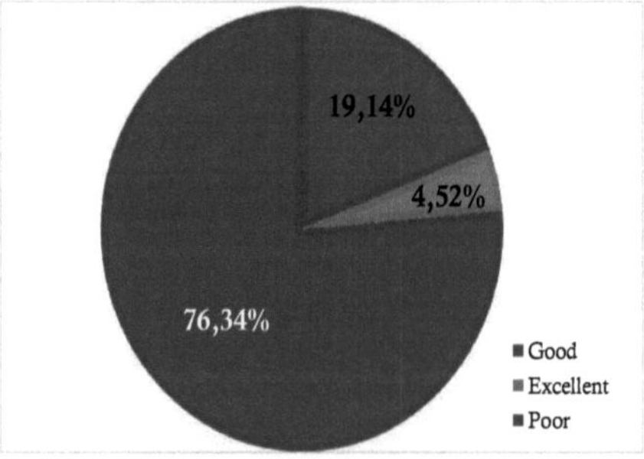

Figure 12. Total knowledge score for respondents on DND

Total knowledge scores were calculated. Overall, 23.66% of the participants had good or perfect knowledge scores.

Table XIII. Demographic and professional characteristics of respondents in relation to their level of knowledge about sickle cell disease.

Variable	Total (N=465)	Bonne connaissance (n=37)		Connaissance insuffisante (n=428)		p-value
Âge (années)						
20-29	151	7	(4,64%)	144	(95,36%)	0,478
30-39	208	22	(10,58%)	186	(89,42%)	0,509
≥40	106	8	(7,55%)	98	(92,45%)	
Sexe						
Féminin	233	15	(6,4%)	218	(93,56%)	0,297
Masculin	232	22	(9,48%)	210	(90,52%)	
Titre médical						
Médecin	204	30	(14,71%)	174	(85,29%)	<0,0001
Infirmier	261	7	(2,68%)	254	(97,32%)	
Type de formation sanitaire						
Publique	309	27	(8,74%)	282	(91,26%)	0,487
Privée	156	10	(6,41%)	146	(93,59%)	
Expérience clinique (années)						
≤5	245	22	(8,98%)	223	(91,02%)	0,491
>5	220	15	(6,12%)	205	(93,18%)	
Formation sur la drépanocytose au cours de 2 dernières années						
Oui	116	11	(9,48%)	105	(90,52%)	0,615
Non	349	26	(7,45%)	323	(92,55%)	

Of the 465 respondents, only 37 (7.96%) had good knowledge (knowledge score ≥8) and 428 others (92.04%) had insufficient knowledge. Nearly 15% of doctors and nearly 3% of nurses had good knowledge of sickle cell disease. The association between medical title and knowledge of sickle cell disease was statistically significant (p<0.0001), indicating that doctors were significantly better informed than nurses. In addition, neither age, sex, type of health facility, number of years of clinical experience, nor the fact of having attended a training session on sickle cell disease had any influence on respondents' level of knowledge (p>0.05).

Table XIV. Demographic and professional characteristics of respondents in relation to their level of knowledge about NHW

Variable	Total N=465	Niveau de connaissance				p-value
		Bon/Excellent (n=110)		Mauvais (n=355)		
Age						
20-29 ans	151	30	(19,87%)	121	(80,13%)	0,278
30-39 ans	208	52	(25,00%)	156	(75,00%)	0,892
≥40 ans	106	28	(26,42%)	78	(73,58%)	
Sexe						
Masculin	232	67	(28,88%)	165	(71,12%)	0,008
Féminin	233	43	(18,45%)	190	(81,55%)	
Titre médical						
Médecin	204	65	(31,86%)	139	(68,14%)	0,0003
Infirmier	261	45	(17,24%)	216	(82,76%)	
Expérience clinique						
≤5 ans	245	53	(21,63%)	192	(78,37%)	0,303
6-10 ans	122	30	(24,59%)	92	(75,41%)	0,731
>10 ans	98	27	(27,55%)	71	(72,45%)	
Séance de formation sur la drépanocytose au cours de 2 dernières années						
Oui	349	84	(24,07%)	265	(75,93%)	0,812
Non	116	26	(22,41%)	90	(77,59%)	
Type de formation sanitaire						
Centre de santé	81	19	(23,46%)	62	(76,54%)	0,228
HGR	163	37	(22,70%)	126	(77,30%)	0,117
Clinique privée	156	32	(20,51%)	124	(79,49%)	0,053
Cliniques Universitaires	65	22	(33,85%)	43	(66,15%)	

Good or excellent total knowledge scores were not significantly related to the following variables: age, type of facility, sickle cell training session and clinical experience. However, male participants were significantly more likely to obtain good or excellent knowledge scores than female participants (p=0.008). With regard to the participants' medical title, the proportion of good or excellent knowledge scores among doctors was statistically higher than among nurses (p=0.0003).

5. Discussion

This study assessed healthcare providers' knowledge of sickle cell disease and its neonatal screening. It is recognised that the level of knowledge is indirectly reflected in the quality of healthcare provided to patients by healthcare providers [24].The results of this study provided a basis on which to develop training sessions on sickle cell disease and neonatal screening for healthcare providers in Lubumbashi. Given that the DRC is the second country in Africa most affected by the disease (after Nigeria), with an estimated prevalence of 2% [6,7], but ranging from 3.47 to 7.1% among newborns in Lubumbashi [8,9], it would be expected that a large number of healthcare providers would have good or excellent knowledge of the disease and its neonatal screening.Several studies assessing the level of knowledge about sickle cell disease have shown that doctors and nurses have insufficient knowledge about this disease

[25]. In general, the study reported 7.96% good knowledge of sickle cell disease and 23.66% good or excellent knowledge of neonatal screening. Mc Walter et al in 2011 in the United States of America (USA) found 89.4% good or perfect knowledge [21]. Concerning the 13 questions on sickle cell anaemia, only in three areas (neonatal screening, definition and genotyping of sickle cell anaemia) did the proportion of professionals giving correct answers reach more than 58%. In the others, the rates of correct answers varied from 11.6% to 46.0%. Nearly two-thirds (64.3%) of participants said that sickle cell disease could be diagnosed by a complete blood count or a red blood cell count. However, with regard to the type of health facility, compared to the health providers in the health facilities public health facilities were significantly more likely to know that the sickle cell disease does not only affect African-American individuals (p=0.035). These results suggest that some topics are not successfully covered or communicated in training sessions and that sickle cell training needs to be done regularly to update healthcare providers in our setting after identifying effective methods and specific content for these sessions. McWalter et al [21] have suggested that the management of patients with anaemia may contribute more to knowledge of sickle cell disease than simply attending education sessions. The low percentage of correct answers given by doctors and nurses to most of the questions asked shows that these professionals have insufficient knowledge to help people with sickle cell disease, leading indirectly to a poor outcome in terms of the assistance they can provide. It follows from this finding that these professionals should be included in the regular learning process about sickle cell anaemia. Doctors and nurses offer great potential in terms of health promotion and preventive action [26]. It is important to note that doctors were significantly more likely than nurses to answer several knowledge questions correctly. However, we found that 14.71% of doctors had significantly more knowledge than nurses (2.68%) about sickle cell disease and 31.86% of doctors compared with 17.24% of nurses about neonatal screening. Similar results were reported by Barroso et al [25]. Nurses are most of the time the first to come into contact with the patient, taking vital signs and supporting the medical diagnosis; they always work with a view to maintaining an interdisciplinary team [25]. This is so as not to delay the patient's care, and so their level of knowledge should be sufficient.The study reported that 75% of professionals had stated that they had not attended a training session on sickle cell disease. This finding is similar to that made by Barroso et al [25], who noted that a large number of professionals had not received training on the subject (94.2%). When the level of knowledge about sickle cell anaemia was compared with the number of years of clinical experience, it was found that there was no statistically significant association. This finding shows that there is an urgent and emerging need to update and train professionals in all aspects of sickle cell disease, focusing on the roles of each professional, with the aim of making an early diagnosis and guiding care to improve the quality of life of patients with sickle cell disease. The results of this knowledge assessment study can be used to identify areas where training programmes need to be intensified [27]. Education based on continuous learning is a necessary condition for the development of the subject in terms of improving care. The search for continuity in the education of healthcare professionals, through postgraduate courses and also free training, must not only be an initiative of the institution to which they are linked, but above all a commitment to each individual aimed at personal, professional and social transformation [25]. This study showed that doctors and nurses in our environment lack sufficient information in the field of sickle cell disease. Brazilian studies have shown that educational interventions

have been effective in increasing the knowledge of healthcare providers [24,26]. It is the responsibility of health authorities to ensure the ongoing training, qualification and education of these professionals during their service [28]. In order to produce satisfactory and effective results to meet the needs generated by the dynamic nature of the problems. One of the limitations of this study, based on closed, self-administered questionnaires, was that participants were allowed to take their time in answering them, so as not to feel that they were being watched by a supervisor. As a result, we could not be sure of the veracity of the answers given by the participants at the time, but out of respect for ethics we trusted the results given that they had expressed their willingness to participate freely in the study. Another selection bias in this study is that by excluding health facilities that did not have a minimum of 50 births per month, some care providers were excluded from the study.

6.Conclusion

This study shows that knowledge gaps exist regarding sickle cell disease and its neonatal screening among health care providers in Lubumbashi. These results suggest opportunities for additional training on sickle cell disease in general to ensure a competent healthcare workforce in an environment highly affected by sickle cell disease.

References

1. Makani J, Ofori-Acquah SF, Nnodu O, Wonkam A, Ohene-Frempong K. Sickle cell disease: new opportunities and challenges in Africa. The Scientific World Journal 2013; 2013: Article ID 193252.
2. Mukuku O, Sungu JK, Mutombo AM, Mawaw MP, Aloni NM, Wemonyama OS and Luboya NO. Albumin, copper, manganese and cobalt levels in children suffering from sickle cell anemia at Kasumbalesa, in Democratic Republic of Congo. BMC Hematol 2018; 18: 23.
3. Bello-Manga H, DeBaun MR, Kassim AA. Epidemiology and treatment of relative anemia in children with sickle cell disease in sub-Saharan Africa. Expert review of hematology 2016; 9(11): 1031-1042.
4. Connes P. Physiopathology of sickle cell disease. In: de Montalembert, Allali S, Brousse V, Marchetti MT. Sickle cell disease in children and adolescents. Paris: Elsevier Masson; 2020.
5. Piel FB, Patil AP, Howes RE, Nyangiri OA, Gething PW et al. Global epidemiology of sickle haemoglobin in neonates: a contemporary geostatistical model-based map and population estimates. Lancet. 2013.
6. Tshilolo L, Aissi LM, Lukusa D, Kinsiama C, Wembonyama S, Gulbis B, Vertongen F. Neonatal screening for sickle cell anemia in the Democratic Republic of the Congo: experience from a pioneer project on 31204 newborns. J Clin Pathol. 2009;62(1):35-8.
7. Agasa B, Bosunga K, Opara A, Tshilumba K, Dupont E, Vertongen F, Cotton F, Gulbis B. Prevalence of sickle cell disease in a northeastern of the Democratic Republic of Congo: What impact on transfusion policy? Transfus Med. 2010 ;20(1) :62-5.
8. Shongo MYP, Mukuku O. Neonatal screening for sickle cell disease in Lubumbashi,

Democratic Republic of Congo. Revue de l'Infirmier Congolais 2018; 2(1): 62-63.

9. Katamea T, Mukuku O, Wembonyama SO. Newborn screening for sickle cell disease in Lubumbashi city, Democratic Republic of the Congo: a preliminary study on an update of the disease prevalence. British Journal of Hematology 2021; 193(S1): 31.

10. Makani J, Cox SE, Soka D, Komba AN, Oruo J, Mwamtemi H, et al. Mortality in Sickle Cell Anemia in Africa: A Prospective Cohort Study in Tanzania. PLoS ONE 2011; 6(2): e14699.

11. Grosse SD, Odame I, Atrash HK, Amendah DD, Piel FB, Williams TN. Sickle cell disease in Africa: a neglected cause of early childhood mortality. American journal of preventive medicine 2011; 41(6): S398-S405.

12. Consensus conference. Newborn screening for sickle cell disease and other hemoglobinopathies. JAMA. 1987;258(9):1205-1209.

13. Ware RE, de Montalembert M, Tshilolo L, Abboud MR. Sickle cell disease. Lancet 2017; 390 (10091): 311-323.

14. Mariane DM, Tshilolo L, Allali S. Sickle cell disease: a comprehensive program of care from birth. Hematology 2019; (1): 490-495.

15. Oyeku SO, Feldman HA, Ryan K, Muret-Wagstaff S, Neufeld EJ. Primary care clinicians' knowledge and confidence about newborn screening for sickle cell disease: randomized assessment of educational strategies. Journal of the National Medical Association 2010 ; 102(8) : 676-683.

16. Diniz KKS, Pagano AS, Fernandes APPC, Reis IA, Pinheiro LG, Torres HDC. Development and validation of an instrument to assess Brazilian healthcare professional providers' knowledge on sickle cell disease. Hematology, transfusion and cell therapy 2019; 41 : 145-152.

17. Kambale-Kombi, P, Marini Djang'eing'a R, Alworong'a OparaJP, Tonen-Wolyec S, Kayembe Tshilumba C, Batina-Agasa S. Students' knowledge on sickle cell disease in Kisangani, Democratic Republic of the Congo. Hematology2020; 25(1): 91-94.

18. Mukinayi BM, Kalenda DK, Mbelu S, Gulbis B. Knowledge and behaviour of 50 Congolese families affected by sickle cell disease: a local survey. The Pan African. Medical Journal 2018; 29: 24.

19. Batina SA, Kambale PK, Sabiti MP, et al. Barriers to health-care for sickle cell disease patients in the Democratic Republic Congo. Afr J Health Issues.2017;1:2.

20. Oyeku SO, Feldman HA, Ryan K, Muret-Wagstaff S, Neufeld EJ. Primary care clinicians' knowledge and confidence about newborn screening for sickle cell disease: randomized assessment of educational strategies. Journal of the National Medical Association 2010 ; 102(8) : 676-683.

21. McWalter KM, White EM, Hayes DK, Au SM. Hemoglobinopathy newborn screening knowledge of physicians. American journal of Preventive Medicine 2011; 41(6): S384- S389.

22. Kemper AR, Uren RL, Moseley KL, Clark SJ. Primary care physicians' attitudes regarding follow-up care for children with positive newborn screening results. Pediatrics. 2006 ;118(5) :1836-1841.

23. DRC Ministry of Public Health. Rapport des comptes de la santé 2014. Kinshasa: PNCNS; October 2016.

24. Gomes LMX, Vieira MM, Reis TC, de Andrade-Brabosa TL, Caldeira AP. Understanding of technical education level professionals regarding sickle cell disease: a descriptive study. Online Brazilian Journal of Nursing 2013; 12(3): 482-490.
25. Barroso LMFM, Araújo TME, Alves BE, de Carvalho MDC. Professional knowledge of the family health strategy on sickle-cell disease. Revista de Pesquisa Cuidado é Fundamental Online 2013; 5(6): 9-19.
26. Gomes LMX, Vieira MM, Reis TC, Andrade-Barbosa TL, Caldeira AP. Knowledge of family health program practitioners in Brazil about sickle cell disease : a descriptive, cross-sectional study. BMC Fam Pract. 2011; 12 (89):1-7.
27. Jenerette CM, Brewer CA, Silva S, Tanabe P. Does attendance at a sickle cell educational conference improve clinician knowledge and attitude toward patients with sickle cell disease? Pain Management Nursing 2016; 17(3): 226-234.
28. Nascimento EPL, Correa CRS. O agente comunitário de saúde: formação, inserção e práticas. Cad saúde pública. 2008 ; 24(6) : 1304-13.

CHAPTER IV
GENERAL DISCUSSION

We propose to conduct the present argument in correlation with the objectives set, those relating to :

Determining the diagnostic reliability of the Sickle SCAN® test in newborn screening in Lubumbashi

Early diagnostic testing remains a key factor in reducing mortality from this disease [1]. The rapid test was able to perfectly detect the Hb AC and Hb SS phenotypes diagnosed by capillary electrophoresis, and the sensitivity is almost perfect for Hb AS and Hb AA. Overall, the proportion of misclassifications (discordant results between Sickle SCAN® and capillary electrophoresis) is estimated at 2.74% (10/365) of the tests performed, a rate higher than the 1.1% found in West Africa (Bamako and Lomé) by Segbena et al [2] and less than 4% of that reported in Paris (France) in the study by Nguyen-Khoa et al [3]. Nwegbu MM et al in 2017 in Nigeria (Gwagwalada) found a mismatch rate of 1.8% compared to high performance liquid chromatography [4].In terms of reliability, the Sickle scan test in our study demonstrated a sensitivity of 95.83% to 100% and a specificity of 96.48% to 100% in the detection of Hb A, Hb S, Hb C compared to electrophoresis as the reference method. Smart LR et al in 2018 similarly in Tanzania (Mwanza) showed a sensitivity of 98.1% and specificity of 91.1% [5]. Mc Gann PT et al in 2016 in the USA (Cincinnati) showed a sensitivity of 98.3% to 100% and a specificity of 92.5% to 100% [6]. Siana N et al in 2019 in Tanzania (Dar es Salaam), found a sensitivity of 100% and a specificity of 98% to 100% [7], Julie K et al in 2015 in South Carolina (Charleston and Durham), found a sensitivity of 100% and a specificity of 98% to 100% [8].

Determine the level of acceptability of DND and the factors influencing it in the population of the city of Lubumbashi

The good acceptability of DND among the Lushois population can be seen with a rate of 84.50 This is relatively close to the 86% found by Oluwole et al (Lagos) [9] and 86.1% found by Nnodu et al [10] in Nigeria. Higher rates have been reported: 99% by Tubman et al [11] in Liberia (Monrovia) and 99.7% by Odunvbun et al [12] in Nigeria (Benin City). In contrast to our results, however, a recent study carried out in Koula-Moutou (Gabon) by Mombo LE et al in 2021 found an acceptability rate of 30% [13]. We believe that our results can be partly explained by the fact that a large majority of the population is Christian. Our results also show that the level of acceptability of DND was associated with age and gender, in contrast to the study by Nnodu et al [10]. However, female respondents were more favourable than male respondents. We believe that this is due to the roles played by African women and their position in the household, as Agnès Lainés also demonstrated in Paris in 2012: "... they are the ones who look after and educate the children, they are also often the financial supporters of their families, the contacts for doctors, they are the ones who attend consultations and often also work in associations... Their burden is as much moral as it is physical or material...".

[14].Compared to Protestants/Pentecostals and Catholics, Muslims were less accepting of DND. This finding is consistent with that of Nnodu et al [10] who found that Muslims were less supportive of DND. We believe this is partly due to the fact that a large majority of Christian churches require couples intending to enter into marriage to be tested beforehand. Only 18.55% of people with sickle cell disease knew their status, a much higher rate than in Nigeria (3.5%), according to Modell B et al in 2007 [15]. This is thought to be due to a lack of awareness and misconceptions that need to be adequately addressed not only at all levels of healthcare, but also through functional intersectoral collaboration, particularly with the media.

Determining the prevalence of sickle cell disease in newborns in Lubumbashi

Nine maternity units in the city of Lubumbashi carried out neonatal screening for sickle cell anaemia in 600 mothers, with a participation rate of 89.7%. The prevalence study found that 5.01% of newborns were SS (homozygous sickle cell), 26.21% were AS (sickle cell trait carriers) and 0.19% were AC (C trait carriers). Before us, Shongo and Mukuku in 2018 found a prevalence of 12.14% Hb AS and 3.47% Hb SS during a survey conducted in 3 health facilities in the city of Lubumbashi [16]. Vierin NY et al in 2012 in Gabon (Libreville) in a study conducted in 2 maternity units found a prevalence of 15.10% Hb AS and 1.80% Hb SS [17]. Agasa et al in 2007 in a study conducted in 5 health facilities in the city of Kisangani, found a prevalence of 23.3% of Hb AS and 0.96% of Hb SS [18] and in another study conducted by Tshilolo et al throughout the DRC in 2009 reported a prevalence of 16.9% of Hb AS and 1.4% of Hb SS [19]. In 2008, Mutesa L et al conducted a study in the Great Lakes region (Burundi, Rwanda and the eastern part of the DRC) in 4 maternity units and found a prevalence of 3.28% of Hb AS and 0.11% of Hb SS [20]. Odunvbun ME et al in 2008 in Nigeria (Benin City), found a prevalence of 20.6% of Hb AS and 2.8% of Hb SS [12]. Siana N et al in 2019 in Tanzania (Dar es Salaam) reported 12.7% Hb AS, 0.8% Hb SS [7]. Antoine LK et al in 2021 in Kindu (DRC) reported a prevalence of 1.9% SS Hb, 26.8% AS Hb [21]. This high prevalence of 5.01% (which increases over time) is thought to be the result of a lack of neonatal screening, population growth, a major lack of knowledge about sickle cell disease among healthcare providers and the lack of an active national programme to combat sickle cell disease.

Assessing health professionals' knowledge of sickle cell disease and neonatal screening in Lubumbashi, Democratic Republic of Congo

We found that 7.96% of the target population in our survey had good knowledge of sickle cell disease, a finding similar to that of Barroso et al in 2013 in Brazil [22]. And 23.66% had good or excellent knowledge of neonatal screening, unlike Mc Walter et al [23] in 2011 in the USA (Hawaii, San Francisco and Salt Lake City) who found 89.4% had good or perfect knowledge. Specifically, more than 58% of correct answers were given, only in three themes on sickle cell anaemia, namely: neonatal screening, definition and genotyping of sickle cell anaemia. In the other themes, the rates of good response varied from 11.6% to 46.0%. Regarding neonatal screening, 64.3% of participants stated that the disease could be diagnosed by a complete blood count or a red blood cell count. In terms of type of health facility, compared with private health facility providers, public health facility providers were significantly more likely to know that sickle cell disease does not affect African-American individuals (74.11%). We also found that 46.57% of doctors had a much higher level of knowledge than nurses (19.92%) about sickle cell disease and neonatal screening. Similar results (29.8% of doctors and 54.4% of nurses) were reported before us by Barroso et al [22]. Our study also reported that 75% of professionals had stated that they had not attended a training session on sickle cell disease. This finding is perfectly comparable to that made by Barroso et al. in Brazil, who noted that a large number of professionals had not received training in sickle cell disease (94.2%) [22]. These results demonstrate a significant lack of knowledge among healthcare providers about sickle cell disease in general.

Limitations of the study :

In the case of the closed, self-administered questions, participants were given the opportunity to take their time in answering them, so as not to feel that they were being watched by a supervisor. As a result, we could not be sure of the veracity of the answers given by the participants at the time, but out of respect for ethics we trusted the results given that they had expressed their willingness to participate freely in the study. A major limitation of the study on the acceptability of DND by the Lush population is the possibility of selection bias, as our study population is exclusively urban. Thus, the results of this study could only be considered applicable to the urbanised population, but the results of this research constitute an acceptable starting point for discussion on a national policy for DND.

References

1. Platt OS, Brambilla DJ, Rosse WF, Milner PF, Castro O, Steinberg MH, et al. Mortality in sickle cell disease. Life expectancy and risk factors for early death 1994. N Engl J Med;330(23):1639-44.
2. Segbena AY, Guindo A, Buono R, Kueviakoe I, Diallo DA, Guernec G, et al. Diagnostic accuracy in field conditions of the sickle SCAN® rapid test for sickle cell disease among children and adults in two West African settings: the DREPATEST study 2018. BMC hematology; 18: 26.
3. Nguyen-Khoa T, Mine L, Allaf B, Ribeil JA, Remus C, Stanislas A, Gauthereau V, Enouz S, Kim JS, Yang X, Gluckman E, Beaudeux JL, Munnich A, Girot R, and Cavazzana M. Sickle SCAN™ (BioMedomics) fulfills analytical conditions for neonatal screening of sickle cell disease 2018. Ann Biol Clin; 76(4): 416-20.
4. Nwegbu MM, Isa HA, Nwankwo BB, Okeke CC, Edet-Offong UJ, Akinola NO et al. Preliminary evaluation of a point-of-care testing device (Sickle SCAN) in screening for sickle cell disease 2017. Hemoglobin.;41(2):77–82.
5. Smart LR, Ambrose EE, Raphael KC, Hokororo A, Kamugisha E, Tyburski EA, Lam WA, Ware RE and McGann PT. Simultaneous point-of-care detection of anemia and sickle cell disease in Tanzania: the RAPID study 2018. Ann Hematol. 97(2):239-46.
6. McGann PT, Schaefer BA, Paniagua M, Howard TA and Ware RE. Characteristics of a rapid, point-of-care lateral flow immunoassay for the diagnosis of sickle cell disease 2016.

Am J Hematol. 91(2):205-10.

7. Siana N, Lillian M, Deogratias S, Vera M, Promise B.M, et al. Newborn screening for sickle cell disease: an innovative pilot program to improve child survival in Dar es Salaam, Tanzania Int Health 2019; 11: 589-595

8. Julie K, Marilyn JT, Carolyn H, Christopher L.R, Jason S. K and Xiaoxi Y. Validation of a novel point of care testing device for sickle cell disease 2015. V 13, N° of article: 225.

9. Oluwole EO, Adeyemo TA, Osanyin GE, Odukoya OO, Kanki PJ and Afolabi BB Feasibility and acceptability of early infant screening for sickle cell disease in Lagos, Nigeria- A pilot study 2020. PLoS ONE 15(12): e0242861.

10. Nnodu OE, Adegoke SA, Ezenwosu OU, Emodi II, Ugwu NI, Ohiaeri CN, et al. A Multi-centre Survey of Acceptability of Newborn Screening for Sickle Cell Disease in Nigeria 2018. Cureus; 10(3): e2354.

11. Tubman VN, Marshall R, Jallah W, Guo D, Ma C, Ohene-Frempong K, et al. Newborn Screening for Sickle Cell Disease in Liberia: A pilot study 2016. Pediatr Blood Cancer; 63 (4): 671-676.

12. Odunvbun ME, Okolo AA, Rahimy CM. Newborn screening for sickle cell disease in a Nigerian hospital 2008. Public health; 122(10): 1111-1116.

13. Mombo LE, Makosso LK, Bisseye C, Mbacky K, Setchell JM and Edou A. Acceptability of neonatal sickle cell disease screening among parturient women at the Paul Moukambi Regional Hospital in rural Eastern Gabon, Central Africa 2021. African Journal of Reproductive Health; 25(3): 72-77.

14. LAINÉ Agnès. "Women as victims? Comprendre la construction d'une anthropologie collective dans des jeux d'échelles face au risque de drépanocytose" 2012. Migrations santé, n° 144-145, pp. 133-162.

15. Modell B, Darlison M. Global epidemiology of haemoglobin disorders and derived service indicators 2008. Bull WHO; 86(6):480-7.

16. Shongo MYP, Mukuku O. Neonatal screening for sickle cell disease in Lubumbashi, DRC 2018. Revue de l'Infirmier Congolais. 2 : 62-63.

17. Vierin Nzame Y, Boussougou Bu Badinga I, Koko J, Blot Ph and Moussavou A. Screening neonatal sickle cell disease in Gabon 2012. Médecine d'Afrique Noire; 59 (2): 95-99.

18. Agasa B, Bosunga K, Opara A, Tshilumba K, Dupont E, Vertongen F, Cotton F, Gulbis B. Prevalence of sickle cell disease in a northeastern region of the Democratic Republic of Congo: what impact on transfusion policy? J Med Screen. 2007; 14(3): 113-6.

19. Tshilolo L, Aissi LM, Lukusa D, Kinsiama C, Wembonyama S, Gulbis B and Vertongen F. Neonatal screening for sickle cell anaemia in the Democratic Republic of the Congo: experience from a pioneer project on 31 204 newborns 2010. Transfus Med ; 20(1) : 62-5.

20. Mutesa L, Boemer F, Ngendahayo L, Rulisa S, Rusingiza EK, Cwinya-Ay N, Mazina D, Kariyo PC, Bours V and Schoos R. Neonatal screening for sickle cell disease in Central Africa: a study of 1825 newborns with a new enzyme-linked immunosorbent assay test 2008. Public Heath; 122(9): 933-41.

21. Antoine LK, Franck NL, Donatien KNN, Léon TM. Neonatal screening for sickle cell disease in the town of Kindu, eastern Democratic Republic of Congo: preliminary study in

nine maternity units, 2021.

22. Barroso LMFM, Araújo TME, Alves BE, de Carvalho MDC. Professional knowledge of the family health strategy on sickle-cell disease 2013. Revista de Pesquisa Cuidado é Fundamental Online; 5(6): 9-19.

23. McWalter KM, White EM, Hayes DK, Au SM. Hemoglobinopathy newborn screening knowledge of physicians. American journal of Preventive Medicine 2011; 41(6): S384- S389.

GENERAL CONCLUSION

At the end of this work, we note that : The Sickle SCAN® test has demonstrated indisputable reliability (97.26%) in DND in Lubumbashi. Given its advantages, it will be highly beneficial and efficient in the overall care of children with sickle cell disease, and will facilitate the implementation of large-scale systematic screening programmes. The acceptability of neonatal screening for sickle cell disease is 84.5% and is influenced by by age, religion and gender.The prevalence of sickle cell disease is high due to the lack of screening measures despite the existence of numerous previous publications. In our study, 68.59% of newborns were AA, 26.21% AS, 5.01% SS and 0.19% AC. In general, 7.96% of healthcare professionals had a good knowledge of sickle cell disease and 23.66% had a good knowledge of DND.

OUTLOOK

To improve the survival of children with sickle cell disease, it would be advisable to :

• Develop training and information programmes to be integrated into the system national education system (primary, secondary and university)

• Tracking screened children longitudinally

RECOMMENDATIONS

In sub-Saharan Africa, sickle cell disease is often diagnosed in late childhood when clinical symptoms first appear. The high cost and complexity of conventional diagnostic methods limit neonatal screening. These methods are neither rapid nor easy to implement in resource-limited settings, as they require substantial financial investment. Our recommendations can be summarised as follows:

1° To the Ministry of Public Health :

❖ Given its low cost, speed and reliability, the Sickle Scan test should be made available in all health zones in order to systematically scale up DND with a view to covering the whole country. This will enable preventive and mass care of sickle-cell anaemic children to be put in place, and will generate national sickle-cell anaemia registers.
❖ Introduce systematic neonatal screening before maternity wards are discharged;

❖ Set up active ongoing training programmes for healthcare staff on sickle cell disease and its management;
❖ Stepping up mass mobilisation and awareness-raising efforts, with appeals to religious leaders and the media to demonstrate the value of premarital screening for sickle cell anaemia.

2° Doctors and nurses working in paediatric medicine

❖ Participate in continuing education programmes on sickle cell anaemia in order to ensure that a skilled health workforce in a highly affected environment.

3° To the Community :

❖ Adhere to the sickle cell screening and management programmes recommended by healthcare staff through awareness-raising campaigns.

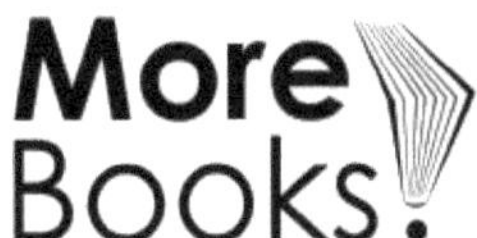

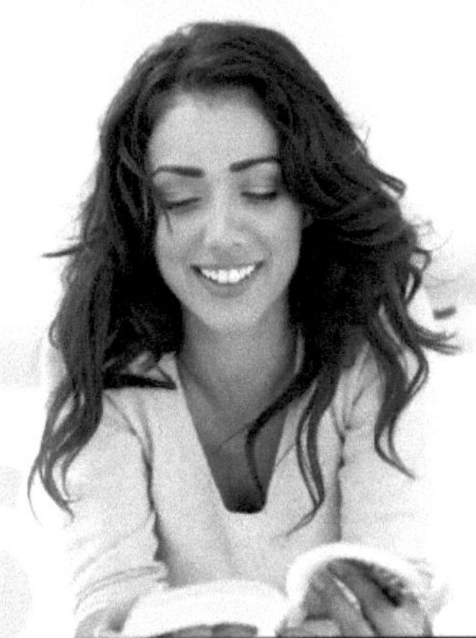

I want morebooks!

Buy your books fast and straightforward online - at one of world's fastest growing online book stores! Environmentally sound due to Print-on-Demand technologies.

Buy your books online at
www.morebooks.shop

Kaufen Sie Ihre Bücher schnell und unkompliziert online – auf einer der am schnellsten wachsenden Buchhandelsplattformen weltweit! Dank Print-On-Demand umwelt- und ressourcenschonend produzi ert.

Bücher schneller online kaufen
www.morebooks.shop

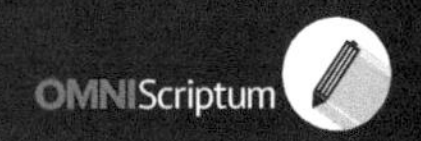

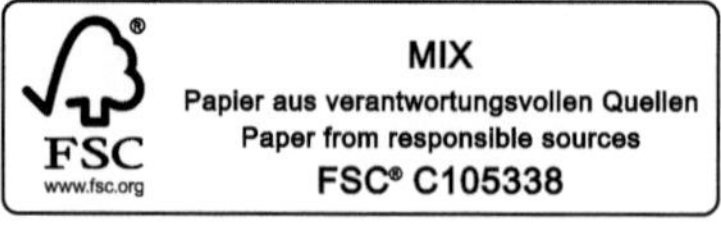

Printed by Books on Demand GmbH, Norderstedt / Germany